Adenomyosis

Min Xue · Jinhua Leng
Felix Wong

Editors

Adenomyosis

Facts and treatments

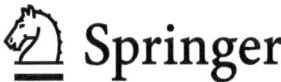 Springer

Editors
Min Xue
Department of Obstetrics and Gynecology
Third Xiangya Hospital
Changsha, China

Jinhua Leng
Department of Obstetrics and Gynecology
Peking Union Medical College Hospital
Beijing, China

Felix Wong
School of Women's and Children's Health
The University of New South Wales
Sydney, Australia

ISBN 978-981-33-4094-7   ISBN 978-981-33-4095-4   (eBook)
https://doi.org/10.1007/978-981-33-4095-4

This Springer imprint is published by the registered company Springer Nature Singapore Pte Ltd.
The registered company address is: 152 Beach Road, #21-01/04 Gateway East, Singapore 189721,
Singapore

Foreword I

Confusion and Puzzle of Adenomyosis Adenomyosis refers to the presence of endometrial glands and stroma in the uterine myometrium. Under the influence of hormones, hyperplasia of the muscle fibers and the connective tissues occurs, forming a diffuse or localized adenomyosis lesion. There is confusion and many puzzles remain unsolved regarding adenomyosis, as well as many ambiguities and disputes. As early as the Hippocrates era 4,000 years ago, there was already a description of adenomyosis; at that time, it was also called "uterine ulcer." In 1860, a German pathologist Carl von Rokitansky simultaneously discovered adenomyosis and endometriosis. At the end of the nineteenth century, adenomyoma was documented in the literature. Thomas Cullen in 1908 further elaborated on the morphology and clinical features of adenomyosis. Sampson in 1927 and Bird in 1972 both gave new definitions of adenomyosis, which have been used up to this day.

This book described the complex and interesting pathogenesis of adenomyosis. Although Sampson's classic pathogenesis theory for endometriosis and adenomyosis is well known, there have been many controversies and doubts about his doctrine. In this book, various theories of pathogenesis are discussed and focused on the latest knowledge including various theories on endometrial invasion, epithelial to mesenchymal cells transformation, Mullerian duct remnants, endometrial stem cell, increased angiogenesis, genetic predisposition, inflammation, and immunological factors as the pathogenesis of adenomyosis.

The diagnosis of adenomyosis is not difficult because of its common symptoms of dysmenorrhea, abnormal uterine bleeding, infertility, etc. These clinical symptoms and their etiologies are individually described in the chapters of this book. After the ultrasound and MRI scans had revealed abnormalities of the endometrial–myometrial interface associated with adenomyosis, people began to explore these noninvasive tools to diagnose adenomyosis. This book describes the various characteristic findings of ultrasound and MRI scans that are very useful for practicing gynecologists to diagnose adenomyosis.

So, this book talks about the various medical and surgical treatments for dysmenorrhea, heavy menstrual bleeding, and infertility. Nevertheless, the conventional treatments are not satisfactory while impacting the reproductive functions and obstetric outcomes of young patients. The treatment of adenomyosis and endometriosis needs to be standardized and long term. An individual treatment plan should be developed for pain, infertility, patient's age, symptoms, disease status, pregnancy wishes, and previous treatment. In 2003 in China, we proposed a treatment policy in 28 Chinese words: remove or eliminate focus, relieve or alleviate pain, restore or promote fertility, and reduce or prevent recurrence. In recent years, more attention to long-term management and comprehensive treatment to protect the patients' bodily functions and quality of life are encouraged. The high-intensity focused ultrasound (HIFU) ablation treatment first described and discussed in this book appears to provide the most appropriate, safe, and potentially long-term management for adenomyosis.

In my opinion, there are still many questions about adenomyosis and endometriosis. The reason why I am relatively brief but a little bit bored in this preface of a book for adenomyosis because adenomyosis is possibly a phenotype of endometriosis to be treated. Both adenomyosis and endometriosis are originally the same kind of disease, and their diagnosis and treatment should be considered as a whole so that they will have a more objective and comprehensive treatment. Of course, this relationship itself can confuse many; those who read this book should bear in mind about targeting treatment to adenomyosis alone because such treatment may not give a satisfactory long-term result.

Professor Felix Wong is a well-known obstetrician and obstetrician and scholar. We have known each other for thirty years, from Hong Kong to Australia. Professor Wong not only devoted himself to academic research and also to clinical work. He had made fruitful contributions to strengthen academic exchanges in mainland China and Hong Kong, and Australia, and even helped develop modern medical and healthcare facilities and talent training in obstetrics and gynecology for China. Professor Wong had coedited some books with Chinese scholars, such as gynecological endoscopy, female genital tract abnormalities, and other reference books in both Chinese and English. This book, which he wrote together with Professor Leng and Professor Xue, is another new contribution.

Best wishes and congratulations!

Lang Jinghe
Chinese Obstetricians and Gynecologists Association
China

Foreword II

Since adenomyosis was proposed as a disease of the uterus in 1908 by Cullen, the increasing use of MRI or ultrasound imaging nowadays on symptomatic patients has contributed to the rising incidence of adenomyosis in the general population. It has also gained more recognition as a difficult disease to provide long-term management. This book discusses the pathogenesis and pathology focusing on trauma, stem cell transformation, genetics, angiogenesis, and humoral factors, all of which have vastly increased the breadth of scientific knowledge as the etiology of adenomyosis. Because more information on adenomyosis has come to light regarding its symptomatology, the authors have separate chapters to discuss these topics, which are very informative. The basic understanding of the pathophysiology of adenomyosis has also led to a shift from solely analgesic medication to appropriate hormonal treatment. In this book, it contains updated information regarding the imaging diagnosis of adenomyosis by ultrasound imaging and MRI. Finally, the authors have not neglected surgical treatment, including the new development of HIFU ablation for the management of this disease.

This book is particularly timely. The need to educate gynecologists and the general public about this disease (adenomyosis) has never been as great because all have to deal with increasing patients with adenomyosis. Many of them have fertility demands and the present medical and surgical treatments have too much adverse impact on their fertility. The focused ultrasound surgery (FUS) mentioned in this book opened up a new world to doctors and patients; it appears to be a favorable noninvasive approach to treat adenomyosis. As with any new treatments, there would be a variation of techniques, and variable results are possible. Sometimes some early results could be disappointing and not up to our desired effect. However, it is hoped that readers can achieve a balanced view of the value and uses of FUS from this book.

It is my wish that when this book is published, it will provide a source of knowledge filling the gap in knowledge for practicing gynecologists, as well as for exploring a new direction of surgical treatment of adenomyosis. Hopefully, it will also stimulate more research in this field to achieve a good outcome of the new treatment.

The authors are to be congratulated for assembling such knowledge on adenomyosis and providing a new solution for adenomyosis treatment. I am particularly glad to write this preface for my friend, Professor Felix Wong, who has collaborated with the Chinese contributors to produce this book for the practicing gynecologists, researchers, and O&G fellows to stimulate their interest in this field of gynecology.

Edward Morris
Royal College of Obstetricians and Gynaecologists,
London, UK

Contents

List of Contributors

Jinhua Leng, MD Department of Obstetrics and Gynecology, Peking Union Medical College Hospital, Beijing, China

Yi Dai, MD Department of Obstetrics and Gynecology, Peking Union Medical College Hospital, Beijing, China

Shan Deng, MD Department of Obstetrics and Gynecology, Peking Union Medical College Hospital, Beijing, China

Xiaoyan Li, MD Department of Obstetrics and Gynecology, Peking Union Medical College Hospital, Beijing, China

Jinghua Shi, MD Department of Obstetrics and Gynecology, Peking Union Medical College Hospital, Beijing, China

Jingjing Lu, MD Department of Radiology/Imaging, Beijing United Family Hospital, Beijing, China

Qing Dai, MD Department of Obstetrics and Gynecology, Peking Union Medical College Hospital, Beijing, China

Guoyun Wang, MD Department of Obstetrics and Gynecology, Qilu Hospital of Shandong University, Jinan, Shandong, China

Min Xue, MD Department of Gynecology and Obstetrics, Third Xiangya Hospital of Central South University, Changsha, Hunan, China

Xiaogang Zhu, MD Department of Gynecology and Obstetrics, Third Xiangya Hospital of Central South University, Changsha, Hunan, China

Mingzhu Ye, MD Department of Gynecology and Obstetrics, Third Xiangya Hospital of Central South University, Changsha, Hunan, China

Can Xie, MD Department of Gynecology and Obstetrics, Third Xiangya Hospital of Central South University, Changsha, Hunan, China

Zhiwen Fan, MD Department of Gynecology and Obstetrics, Third Xiangya Hospital of Central South University, Changsha, Hunan, China

Fang Xiao, MD Department of Gynecology and Obstetrics, Third Xiangya Hospital of Central South University, Changsha, Hunan, China

About the Editors

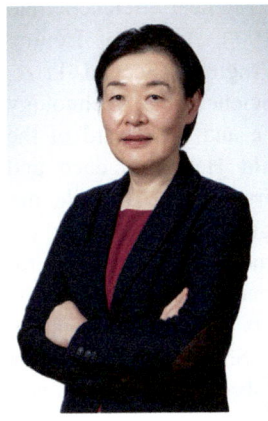

Min Xue is the Professor, Chief Physician, and Doctoral supervisor at the Department of Gynecology and Obstetrics, Third Xiangya Hospital of Central South University. Her main interests are gynecologic endoscopy and gynecological oncology. She was awarded the titles of Xiangya famous doctor and famous doctor of Hunan Province and obtained the Special Government Allowances of the State Council, China.

She is a Standing Committee Member of the Chinese Obstetricians and Gynecologists Association (COGA), Vice-Chairman of Minimally and Non-invasive Medical Association; Member of the Chinese Society of Gynecological Oncology; Chairman of Hunan Obstetrics and Gynecology Association; and Vice-Chairman of Hunan perinatal medicine Association. She is also an Editorial Board Member of *Journal of Practical Gynecology and Obstetrics*, *Journal of Chinese Physician*, *China Journal of Endoscopy*, and the *Journal of Central South University* (Medical Sciences). Her research activities include 5 National research projects and 20 Provincial research projects. She has compiled 21 books and published more than 170 medical papers.

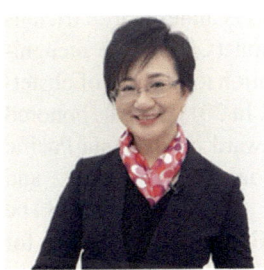

Jinhua Leng MD, is the Professor at the Department of OB/GYN, Peking Union Medical College Hospital, China. She has a clinical practice focusing on complex gynecologic disorders such as endometriosis and adenomyosis. She is also the lead and director for minimally invasive surgery. She holds many other academic positions, including the Chairman of Endometriosis society, Chinese Medical Doctor Association, the Chairman of the Professional Committee of

Endometriosis of Chinese Obstetricians and Gynecologists Association (COGA), the Deputy Chairman of the Laparoscopy Group of Gynecological Minimal Invasive Surgery, the Deputy Head of the Gynecologic Endoscopy Group, COGA, and the Director of Grade 4 Endoscopy Center of the National Health and Family Planning Commission. She was also awarded several prizes for her scientific work, including the Award of National Science and Technology Progress (Second Prize, 2004), Award of Beijing Science and Technology Progress (First Prize, 2006), Award of China Medical Science and Technology (First Prize, 2011), Award of Beijing Science and Technology Progress (Second Prize, 2011), Award of Beijing Science and Technology Progress (Third Prize, 2011), and the Award of the National Maternal and Child Health Science and Technology Achievement (First Prize, 2016). She has published several clinical guidelines including the Chinese Guidelines of Diagnosis and Treatment for Endometriosis (2015) and for adenomyosis (2020) and a consensus of Chinese experts on long-term management of endometriosis (2018). She has published more than 130 papers at home and abroad as the first or corresponding author up to 2020.

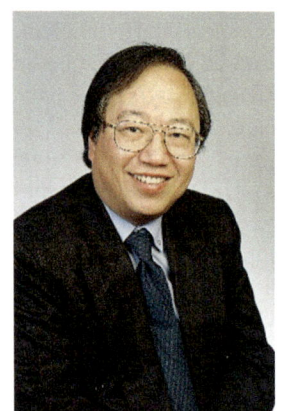

Felix Wong is at present an Adjunct Professor at the University of New South Wales after he retired from his jobs as the past Professor and Medical Director of Liverpool Hospital in Sydney, Australia. He contributed to medical education in Asia Pacific Countries over the past 30 years. In recognition of his contributions to teaching, he received many awards and honors. In 2009, he received the Endos Award in Medical Science and Technology, China, for his excellent achievement in endoscopic surgery. In 2017, he was granted Lin Qiaozhi Cup by the Chinese Obstetricians and Gynecologists Association (COGA) in recognition of his significant contribution to the field of obstetrics and gynecology in China. In 2017, he was honored by Lifetime Achievements Award by the Asia-Pacific Association for Gynecologic Endoscopy and Minimally Invasive Therapy (APAGE). In 2018, he was awarded by the European Society for Gynecological Endoscopy (ESGE) for Outstanding

Contribution Award. Professor Wong had edited 14 medical books and had published more than 200 papers in local and international journals. He is currently the Chairman of the China-Asia Pacific Association of Minimally Invasive Gynecologic Oncologists (CA-AMIGO) and Foundation Chairman of the China-Australia-Asia Pacific Forum of Minimally Invasive Surgery and Vice President of the World Association of Chinese Obstetricians and Gynecologists.

Despite his endoscopic contributions, he continues to contribute toward the development of HIFU education and services in China and Asia Pacific Areas.

The Incidence and Clinical Impact of Adenomyosis

1

Zhiwen Fan

With the advancement of imaging technology, such as ultrasound, more and more patients with asymptomatic adenomyosis are diagnosed, so the incidence of adenomyosis is higher than traditionally thought [1]. An epidemiological study from healthcare institutes in Italy had found that the incidence of adenomyosis in women of reproductive age was 0.02–0.03%, and the prevalence was 0.17% [2]. A cohort study in the United States observed 330,000 women for 10 years and found that the total incidence of adenomyosis in women aged 16–60 years was 1%. The study also found that black women had the highest incidence, while Asian women had the lowest incidence, and white women were somewhere in between [3]. From the literature, there were wide variations in the incidence and prevalence of adenomyosis, and it might be due to the difficulties in accurately assessing the incidence [4–6]. Firstly, there was selection bias in women with indications for a hysterectomy or surgery when this disease was being diagnosed. Secondly, there was a lack of consensus of histological criteria to diagnose adenomyosis, raising concerns about the reproducibility of its histological diagnosis. Thirdly, the increasing use of MRI or ultrasound imaging on symptomatic patients to diagnose this disease without histological confirmation contributed to the increasing incidence in the general population. Nevertheless, the incidence of adenomyosis is related to the patient's age, the number of pregnancy, and pelvic endometriosis.

The incidence of adenomyosis is relatively higher in certain populations, such as 20% of those seeking treatment for various gynecological diseases. Among people with infertility, the incidence of adenomyosis in women over 40 years old is relatively higher, about 30%, and the incidence of adenomyosis in women under 40 years old is about 22% [7].

Z. Fan (✉)
Department of Gynecology and Obstetrics, Third Xiangya Hospital of Central South University, Changsha, Hunan, China

© The Author(s), under exclusive license to Springer Nature Singapore Pte Ltd. 2021
M. Xue et al. (eds.), *Adenomyosis*, https://doi.org/10.1007/978-981-33-4095-4_1

1

1.1   The Clinical Impact of Adenomyosis

1. Dysmenorrhea is a typical symptom of adenomyosis [8]. About 2/3 of the patients may have secondary progressive dysmenorrhea. With time, the degree of pain in the lower abdomen gradually increases as menstrual cramps, the pain duration gradually extends, and even unbearable pain appears. Later, the patient may also experience lower abdominal pain during non-menstrual periods, that is, chronic pelvic pain. If it is associated with pelvic endometriosis, the patient will experience more pain during the non-menstrual period. In addition to the symptoms of dysmenorrhea, 7–10% of patients with adenomyosis can also experience clinical symptoms, such as pain at sexual intercourse (dyspareunia) and persistent pelvic pain.

2. Abnormal uterine bleeding is a common symptom of adenomyosis [8]. About 40–50% of adenomyosis can be manifested as increased menstrual flow, prolonged menstruation, and vaginal spotting before and after menstruation. Still, the most common menstrual abnormality is excessive menstruation, and this can cause anemia to severe patients. It is related to the increase of uterine volume, the increase of the endometrial area of the uterine cavity, and the influence of adenomyosis lesions on the contraction of uterine muscle fibers.

3. Uterine enlargement is an inherent sign of adenomyosis [8]. The uterus may be focally or uniformly enlarged. The gynecological examination can often feel the uniformity of the enlarged uterus, which is spherical, or there is a limited nodular bulge, which is hard and tender, and the menstrual tenderness is obvious.

4. Reduced fertility is also a clinical manifestation of patients with adenomyosis [9]. It is reported in the literature that more than 20% of patients with adenomyosis have infertility. The mechanism may be related to abnormal free radical concentration in the uterine cavity, increased cell inflammation and vascular factors, abnormal uterine contraction, abnormal gene regulation, abnormal embryo implantation, intrauterine membrane abnormality, and tolerance changes, immune abnormalities and changes in adhesion molecules and so on. In addition to adenomyosis with infertility, the probability of a miscarriage, premature delivery, and stillbirth after gestation is significantly higher in patients with adenomyosis than in patients without adenomyosis. Besides, the adverse pregnancy outcomes of patients with adenomyosis, including premature rupture of membranes, preeclampsia, abnormal fetal position, placental abruption, and placenta previa, are also significantly higher than those of non-adenomyosis patients. In recent years, the incidence of adenomyosis with infertility has shown an increasing trend, and low fertility has received increasing attention.

5. Other clinical effects of adenomyosis [8]. Uterine enlargement can cause pressure symptoms by compressing adjacent organs, such as bladder compression can cause urethral symptoms; bowel compression can cause irritable bowel symptoms or constipation. Menorrhagia can lead to anemia. Long-term pain symptoms and infertility can cause mentally and psychologically induced physical disorders.

References

1. Peric H, Fraser I. The symptomatology of adenomyosis. Best Pract Res Clin Obstet Gynaecol. 2006;20(4):547–55.
2. Morassutto C, et al. Incidence and estimated prevalence of endometriosis and adenomyosis in Northeast Italy: a data linkage study. PLoS One. 2016;11(4)
3. Onchee Y, et al. Adenomyosis incidence, prevalence and treatment: United States population – based study 2006–2015. Am J Obstet Gynecol. 2020;223(1):94.e1–94.e10.
4. Chrysostomou M, et al. Incidence of adenomyosis uteri in a Greek population. Acta obstetricia et gynecologica Scandinavica. 1991;70(6):441–4.
5. Raju GC, et al. Adenomyosis uteri: a study of 416 cases. Aust N Z J Obstet Gynaecol. 1988;28(1):72–3.
6. Bird CC, McElin TW, Manalo-Estrella P. The elusive adenomyosis of the uterus—revisited. Am J Obstet Gynecol. 1972;112(5):583–93.
7. Naftalin J, et al. How common is adenomyosis? A prospective study of prevalence using transvaginal ultrasound in a gynaecology clinic. Hum Reprod. 2012;27(12):3432–9.
8. Gordts S, Grimbizis G, Campo R. Symptoms and classification of uterine adenomyosis, including the place of hysteroscopy in diagnosis. Fertil Steril. 2018;109(3):380–388.e1.
9. Harada T, et al. The impact of adenomyosis on women's fertility. Obstet Gynecol Surv. 2016;71(9):557.

The Pathogenesis of Adenomyosis

2

Fang Xiao

Adenomyosis refers to an estrogen-dependent gynecological benign disease in which the endometrial glands and stroma invade the myometrium, resulting in localized or diffuse adenomyosis. It often combines with uterine fibroids, endometrial polyps, endometriosis, etc. The incidence of adenomyosis ranges from 1 to 70% [1] due to the variation of diagnostic criteria. The main clinical manifestations are progressive dysmenorrhea, chronic pelvic pain, menorrhagia, and infertility. With the improvement of magnetic resonance imaging (MRI), transvaginal ultrasound imaging, and other examination techniques, the detection rate of adenomyosis is also increasing [2, 3]. Although it has been nearly 100 years since the name of the disease is mentioned, the true pathogenesis of adenomyosis is still a mystery. This chapter will discuss and focus on the latest knowledge in the pathogenesis of adenomyosis.

2.1   Endometrial Invasion (Into the Myometrium) Theory

The theory of endometrial invasion into the myometrium is also called the basal endometrium invagination theory. Due to the lack of submucosa, the endometrium and the myometrial layers are in direct contact, and the barrier is relatively weak. The junction between the endometrium and the myometrium is called the endometrial-myometrial junctional zone (JZ), and some scholars call it the endometrial myometrial interface (EMI) [4]. Studies have shown that the thickness of JZ in patients with adenomyosis increased significantly. At present, most scholars believe that the thickness of JZ has to exceed 12 mm to diagnose adenomyosis [1, 5].

F. Xiao (✉)
Department of Gynecology and Obstetrics, Third Xiangya Hospital of Central South University, Changsha, Hunan, China

© The Author(s), under exclusive license to Springer Nature Singapore Pte Ltd. 2021
M. Xue et al. (eds.), *Adenomyosis*, https://doi.org/10.1007/978-981-33-4095-4_2

2.1.1 Endometrial Basal Layer Injury

Research studies found that women with a history of uterine or uterine cavity surgery, such as cesarean section, multiple births, multiple abortions, hysteroscopic myomectomy, diagnostic curettage, intrauterine device placement, etc., had almost 1.5 times the incidence of adenomyosis than those without such operations [5, 6]. Therefore these surgical procedures are high-risk factors for the formation of adenomyosis. The surgical operation of the uterus and uterine cavity can cause endometrium and EMI damage. The tissue injury and repair (TIAR) mechanism is activated, and the functional layer of the endometrium is recessed inward through the EMI; it gradually invades the myometrium and leads to the formation of adenomyosis [7]. In pregnancy, it is believed that the proliferation of uterine myocytes, the expansion of the uterine wall, and the involution of the postpartum uterus may damage the endometrium-myometrium JZ, resulting in the invasion of the endometrium into the myometrium.

On the other hand, obstetric complications, such as placental implantation, placental adhesions, uncoordinated uterine contractions, prolonged labor, cesarean section, and gynecological uterine surgery, such as laparoscopic myomectomy, hysteroscopic myomectomy, and endometrial ablation, can directly damage the EMI. Any uterine cavity surgery, like dilatation and curettage (D&C), polypectomy, and surgical abortion, may directly cause gaps or channels between the endometrium and the myometrium, resulting in the invasion of endometrium directly into the myometrium. Besides, adenomyosis is often accompanied by reproductive tract malformations, such as uterine malformation and vaginal septum. These two conditions lead to obstruction of menstrual flow and increase intrauterine pressure, and then it may cause the endometrium to invade into the muscle layer. Finally, congenital developmental abnormalities of the uterus may also have loose connections or gaps between the endometrium and myometrium, which can cause the endometrium to invade the myometrium and cause adenomyosis directly.

2.1.2 Enhancement of Endometrial Invasion and Adhesion Ability Theory

Matrix metalloproteinases (MMP) are a class of enzymes that degrade the extracellular matrix. It is suggested that the overexpression of endometrial metalloproteinase can enhance the endometrial tissue's invasiveness. Li et al. 2006 [8] found that there were high expressions of MMP 2, 3, and 9 in eutopic endometrial and ectopic endometrial tissues in patients with adenomyosis. Their expression levels were significantly higher than those in patients without adenomyosis, and MMP inhibitory enzymes −1 and 2− in endometrial tissue of adenomyosis were significantly lower than the endometrium in those without adenomyosis. Under the influence of various environmental or hormonal factors, the endometrial tissue itself may degrade the extracellular matrix components, including the basement membrane; thereby it can destroy the natural barrier that prevents the endometrium from invading the myometrium, resulting in the formation of adenomyosis.

Cell adhesion molecules are membrane glycoprotein molecules that mediate the interaction between cells or between cells and substrates. They are involved in cell signaling and play an important role in the growth and differentiation of cells, cell migration, tumor metastasis, and wound healing. The expression of cell adhesion molecule-1 in the endometrium and the ectopic endometrium of the uterus with adenomyosis is significantly higher than that without adenomyosis. In addition to cell adhesion molecules, integrin β3 also plays a vital role in the process of cell invasion and adhesion. It not only connects cells and extracellular matrix but also regulates the occurrence of this process through signal transmission and reception. Xiao et al. 2013 [9] also found that the expression level of integrin β3 in the uterine endometrium is lower than that of the ectopic endometrium and uterine endometrium of the uterus without adenomyosis. The integrin expression level of the endometrium in a uterus with adenomyosis is reduced, which can destroy endometrial stability and decrease the basal adhesion of the basal layer, making it easier for the endometrium to invade the myometrium and eventually form the adenomyosis.

2.1.3 Abnormal JZ Between Endometrium and Myometrium

The endometrium-myometrium JZ was first proposed by Hricak H and others in 1983 when they initially used MRI to examine the female reproductive system [10]. Endometrium-myometrium JZ is a new uterine JZ which is different from the JZ in other tissues in the human body, and it lacks an identifiable protective layer – the submucosa. That is, there is no "intermediate buffer zone" between the endometrium and the myometrium, so they are in direct contact. JZ is a special functional unit, which has the functions of regulating trophoblast invasion, providing nutrition, facilitating sperm transport, menstrual hemostasis, and local immunity and is of great significance for maintaining the physiological function of the uterus.

In recent years, with the in-depth study of the pathogenesis of adenomyosis, it has been confirmed that the interface between the endometrium and myometrium is unique, regardless of whether it is structural, functional, histopathological, and by imaging. It plays a key role in the pathogenesis of adenomyosis. The uterine JZ is an estrogen-progestin-dependent transformation zone and shows periodic changes [11]. The embryonic origin of the subendometrial muscle layer is the same as the endometrium, and the anatomical structure is directly connected to the endometrium, so it is speculated that its biological function may be related to the endometrium. In adenomyosis, probably due to the overproduction of estrogen, it may promote oxytocin-mediated uterine activity, causing endometrial hyperplasia and peristaltic enhancement, thereby increasing mechanical stress and tension, chronic long-term abnormalities, and excessive uterine creeping movement may cause micro damage to JZ and activate self-renewing tissue damage repair mechanisms [7, 12, 13].

The activation of the JZ TIAR mechanism promotes the local production of interleukin-1 (IL-1) and induces the activation of COX-2, leading to the production of prostaglandin E2. The steroidogenic acute regulatory protein and cytochrome P450 aromatase are subsequently activated; androgen is formed and aromatized into estrogen, resulting in a high estrogen status in the endometrium. Estrogen acts through estrogen receptors (ER-β) to promote proliferation and healing. During the normal healing process in the normal endometrium, the increase in estrogen secretion gradually stops. However, in the uterus with adenomyosis, the high levels of estrogen stimulate oxytocin-mediated peristalsis through the ER-α receptor, inhibiting the healing process. A positive feedback mechanism is then generated; through which the chronic peristalsis in JZ promotes repeated cycles of injury and repair, resulting in the continuous rupture or damage of muscle fibers in the muscle wall. As each cycle gets worsen, the basal layer of the endometrium enters the myometrium, which eventually leads to the formation of adenomyosis [12, 13]. Also, a large number of studies have shown that abnormal amplitude, frequency, and direction of JZ contraction, especially active peristalsis or sluggish peristalsis, may be the cause of adenomyosis, endometriosis, and infertility [14]. Liu et al. 2013 [15] speculated that the up-regulation of NO (nitric oxide) in smooth muscle cells in the endometrium-myometrium JZ of patients with adenomyosis might be related to the abnormal contractile function of this site. Normal women's uterine contraction during menstrual period is from the fundus of the uterus to the cervix. This contraction helps hemostasis during the menstrual period and helps the exfoliated endometrial tissues exit the uterine cavity. Among patients with adenomyosis, this contraction movement during menstrual period is significantly reduced or not active at all. This abnormal movement makes menstrual blood more easily refluxed into the abdominal cavity, causing endometriosis, which can also explain the high association of adenomyosis and pelvic endometriosis.

2.1.4   The Proliferation of Ectopic Endometrial Cells and Unbalanced Apoptosis: [16]

Uterine adenomyosis is considered to be a proliferative disease. Therefore, the endometrial tissue proliferation ability and the inhibition of apoptosis have attracted much attention. Telomerase is a unique ribonucleoprotein. Its activity continuously adds telomere deoxyribonucleic acid (DNA)-repeating sequence at the end of chromosomes to prevent the loss of telomeres and make cells proliferate and immortalized. It is suggested that the ectopic endometrial cells of patients with adenomyosis under the activation of telomerase can enhance the proliferation ability of ectopic endometrial cells invading the uterine myometrium, promoting the proliferation of surrounding cells and participating in the formation of adenomyosis [16]. In adenomyosis, the expression level of telomerase is significantly higher than other tissues, and the expression level of telomerase in the lesions of severe diffuse adenomyosis is significantly higher than that of a local or mild adenomyosis.

Ki67 is a cell proliferation marker that is expressed only in the nucleus of circulating proliferating cells, not at resting cells. The expression of Ki67 in the ectopic endometrial glandular epithelium of adenomyosis was found to be significantly higher than the control group. It was also higher than that of the normal uterine endometrium in the secretory phase [17]. Besides, Xue et al. 2003 showed that markers related to the proliferation of adenomyosis, such as proliferating cell nuclear antigen, cyclin-1, and cyclin-dependent kinase transfer growth factor and epidermal growth factor, were up-regulated. It suggested that after the endometrial cells invaded the myometrium, their proliferative capacity was enhanced and was important in the development of adenomyosis.

B-cell lymphoma-2 gene (Bcl-2) is called the apoptotic suppressor gene, and survivin protein is an apoptosis-inhibiting protein. Survivin gene is the strongest apoptosis-inhibiting gene currently found. It can exert anti-apoptosis by directly inhibiting the apoptosis pathway. High expression of survivin can promote cell proliferation, participate in the regulation of cell mitosis, and resist various apoptosis-inducing factors, such as interleukin (interleukin, IL) -3, tumor necrosis factor (TNF) -α, chemotherapy, and radiation. The ectopic endometrial tissue of patients with adenomyosis showed a high expression of Bcl-2 and survivin [18], and the two showed a positive correlation. At the same time, Bax has an antagonistic role in the formation and progression of adenomyosis. Its level is down-regulated in the ectopic endometrial tissue in adenomyosis; thus, this leads to enhanced apoptosis inhibition, reduced apoptosis, and increased cell proliferation, participating in the pathogenesis of adenomyosis. Clinical applications of mifepristone and gonadotropin-releasing hormone analog (GnRHa) treatment can reduce levels of Bcl-2 and survivin expression.

Osteopontin (OPN) is a matricellular protein implicated in the pathogenesis of a variety of diseases. It also has an apoptosis-inhibiting effect. If OPN is lacking, the number of cell apoptosis increases significantly. The expression of OPN in the ectopic endometrium of patients with adenomyosis [19] is significantly higher than that of the control group, resulting in the enhanced anti-apoptosis ability of ectopic endometrial cells; thereby they are more likely to survive, and grow. Therefore abnormal apoptosis may be an important factor in the development of adenomyosis.

2.2 Epithelial to Mesenchymal Cells Transformation

Migration and invasion factors are considered to be the key factors for the progression of adenomyosis. Epithelial-mesenchymal transition (EMT) is when epithelial cells lose their cell polarity and become mesenchymal cells to improve their ability to migrate, invade, and resist apoptosis [20, 21]. There are many EMT inducer involved in the process of EMT, and they are E-cadherin, CK7 (an epithelial cell marker), and transforming growth factor-β [22–24]. Chen et al. 2010 [25] found that changes in EMT markers were related to serum E2 levels. Estrogen induced EMT of ER-positive endometrial cells, causing them to migrate and invade. Therefore induced EMT of endometrial epithelial cells contributes to the development of adenomyosis.

From the embryonic development, the mesoderm mesenchyme of the urogenital system transforms into the epithelium to form the endometrium in a specific micro-environment. Mesenchymal epithelialization is not only the direct basis of endometriosis stem cell theory but can also be the direct basis of adenomyosis via EMT. The process of EMT involves a series of important protein molecules and signal transduction pathways, as discussed above. It is currently a hot research topic for endometriosis and adenomyosis. Since the role of the EMT process in the pathogenesis of adenomyosis is still unclear, further research is important.

2.3 Differentiation of Embryonic Multipotent Müllerian Duct Remnant

The Müllerian duct is the original embryonic structure that develops into the female uterus, fallopian tube, and upper vagina during fetal life [26]. The Müllerian duct is composed of surface epithelium and urogenital crest mesenchyme and can differentiate into endometrial glands and stroma [27]. It is speculated that the differentiation of the embryonic pluripotent Müllerian duct remnant in the uterine wall of adult females may lead to the establishment of ectopic endometrial tissue, forming the adenomyosis.

Adenomyosis has the typical characteristics of smooth muscle hyperplasia and fibrosis. In contrast, deep infiltrating endometriotic nodules are also considered to be a possible result of Müllerian duct differentiation, such as proposed by Dunnez et al. 1996 [28]. Adenomyoma and vaginal and rectal septum endometriosis are considered to be extrauterine adenomyosis lesions. They are similar to adenomyosis lesions in pathology and clinical characteristics, and it seems to support this pathogenesis theory.

It is reported in the literature that some patients with congenital genital tract malformation, mayer-rokitansky-küster-hauser (MRKH) syndrome, with their primordial uterus without a functional endometrium, can develop adenomyosis [29]. The finding in these patients did not support the theory of endometrial damage and invasion to explain the occurrence of adenomyosis. Therefore, some scholars proposed that adenomyosis could be developed from the remnant of the Müllerian ducts in the muscular layer.

2.4 Endometrial Stem Cell Theory

Gargett, 2007 [30], had found that there were very few epithelial and mesenchymal stem cells in the endometrium of adult women. Under normal circumstances, endometrial stem cells are at rest. Endometrial stem cells are located in the basal layer of the endometrium. After abnormal shedding, they can enter the pelvis through the fallopian tubes to form endometriosis. If endometrial stem cells migrate abnormally and invade the myometrium, then they form the adenomyosis. Chan et al. 2004 [31] had identified active epithelial and mesenchymal stem cell populations from the basal layer of the endometrium and stroma from hysterectomy specimens. Kato, 2012 [32], confirmed that these stem cells were located among the basal cells of the endometrium and were responsible for the periodic repair of the endometrium after menstruation. In a normal endometrium, the presence of endometrial basal cells is a key factor for regeneration and renewal. However, it can also grow indefinitely and can even extend beyond the endometrium. Some scholars have found that under the stimulation of tissue damage, endometrial stem cells were activated, and proliferation, regeneration, and differentiation occurred, which could promote the invasion as ectopic endometrium. This phenomenon can also be explained by the "stem cell niche hypothesis"; that is to say, the stem cells are located in the niche, and under normal circumstances, the niche can prevent stem cells from proliferating, differentiating, and apoptotic, leaving them in a quiescent state. When the niche is destroyed, stem cells will proliferate, regenerate, and differentiate to varying degrees [33]. The activation of stem cells does not only promote tissue repair, and excessive activation can even lead to the occurrence of proliferative diseases, such as tumors. Therefore, the abnormal activation of endometrial stem cells may be one of the pathogenesis of adenomyosis.

In 2004, Taylor [34] found a donor-derived endometrial gland and mesenchymal cells in the endometrium of four female recipients who received HLA-unmatched bone marrow transplantation, which suggested that bone marrow stem cells could differentiate into endometrial cells. In mice and in vitro experiments [35–37], it also confirmed that bone marrow stem cells could indeed differentiate into mature endometrial cells. From these studies, it can be speculated that bone marrow stem cells may play a role in the development of adenomyosis.

Using electron microscopy, Ibrahim et al. 2015 [38] described another population of stem cells. These stem cells were located in the epithelial glands of the basal endometrium. Because their cytoplasm was electronically glowing, they were called pale cells. In the JZ of patients with adenomyosis, these stem cells were significantly less connected to the surrounding epithelial cells (loss of desmosome junctions). They presented more feet-like structures than in disease-free women. Therefore, it is suggested that in adenomyosis, pale cells might be displaced through the basement membrane, gain movement characteristics, and migrate to the interstitium and then transfer into the myometrium, where they formed new adenomyosis. Pale cell migration requires multiple signaling pathways and biological factors to co-regulate; the cell-to-cell tight connection junction is disintegrated, the expression of adhesion molecules is down-regulated; the basement membrane microrupture and the up-regulation of MMP may be involved in the migration process [39].

2.5 Abnormal Uterine Nerve

Under normal circumstances, the uterine nerves consist of sympathetic and parasympathetic nerves from S2 to S4. These nerve fibers pass through the uterosacral ligament to the paracervical tissue before entering the uterus and form the

Frankenhauser plexus at the posterolateral part of the cervix; the other part of inner-vation is introduced through the other ligaments of the uterus and the peritubal nerve fibers. Most of the uterine nerves are distributed at the interface of the endometrium and myometrium, that is, the nerve distribution in the inner 1/3 of the uterus is greater than the nerve distribution in the outer 2/3, and the nerve can reach the endometrial glandular epithelium and spiral arterioles. Due to the cyclical shrinkage of the endometrial function layer, the nerve fibers on this layer would have periodic denervation and nerve regeneration.

When various factors, such as pregnancy, miscarriage, childbirth, surgery, and infection, cause damage to the uterine nerves, the damaged nerves can release vari-ous neurotransmitters and neural mediators and can attract macrophages and release prostaglandins to the injured area, resulting in the accumulation of inflammatory factors and growth factors. Patients with adenomyosis who show clinical pain symptoms have a large number of abnormal nerve fiber hyperplasias at the interface of the endometrium and myometrium [40]. The abnormal nerve fibers are directly related to the patient's pain and thus involved in the mechanism of pain. These nerve injury and regeneration activities at the JZ may account for the abnormal contrac-tion of the muscular layer and the increase of peristalsis in the JZ in adenomyosis, thus causing other symptoms of adenomyosis.

After treatment with hormonal drugs, such as oral contraceptives, progesterone or levonorgestrel intrauterine system (LNG-IUS), and GnRHa for adenomyosis, in addition to the decrease in nerve fibers in the uterine endometrium and myome-trium, the expression of nerve growth factor (NGF) and its receptors also decreased. Therefore the symptoms of dysmenorrhea improved [41]. On the other hand, estro-gen can increase the expression level of NGF in adenomyosis, thus increasing the severity of adenomyosis. Locally released NGF can stimulate the release of inflam-matory mediators, such as serotonin, histamine, and tumor necrosis factor, by stim-ulating mast cell degranulation, thereby inducing inflammation. It has been shown that increased expression levels of NGF and its receptors in the ectopic endome-trium of adenomyosis can increase the sensitivity of uterine nerves, aggravate the inflammatory response, and cause abnormal growth of local nerve fiber prolifera-tion in adenomyosis. NGF can, in turn, stimulate the expression and release of focal neuropeptides to excite the neuron ends, to maintain the survival and development of sensory neurons, and participate in pain regulation, thus increasing pain or hyper-algesia in adenomyosis. Therefore, abnormal growth of uterine nerve fibers not only participates in the pathogenesis of adenomyosis but also participates in the mecha-nism of dysmenorrhea in adenomyosis.

2.6   The Theory of Increased Angiogenesis

Adenomyosis is often associated with endometrial proliferation, where the growth of endometrial cells requires blood vessels to provide nutrition and eliminate meta-bolic waste. When hysteroscopy is performed on patients with adenomyosis and about 50% of patients have abnormal vascularization in the endometrium [42].

Vascular endothelial growth factor (VEGF) is an important factor that promotes angiogenesis, and its expression level in tissues can reflect tissue angiogenesis. Mu et al. 2014 [43] had shown that in patients with adenomyosis, the number and activity of VEGF in the intima and serum were significantly higher than in normal people, and the level of VEGF in the serum of patients after surgical treatment was reduced compared with before treatment. Compared with a control group, the microvessel density (MVD) in the ectopic endometrium of patients with adenomyosis was significantly increased. Therefore, it can be speculated that the formation of new blood vessels affects the occurrence of adenomyosis, and it may also be the cause of menorrhagia. Liu et al. 2016 [44] found that platelets accumulated in patients with adenomyosis activated the TGF-β1/Smad3 signaling pathway, inducing EMT, fibroblast to myofibroblast transdifferentiation, smooth muscle cell proliferation, and fibrosis and then participated in the development of adenomyosis. Antiplatelet therapy is a potential treatment for adenomyosis, because angiogenesis is a necessary condition for the endometrium to invade the myometrium and continue to grow. The formation of blood vessels not only supplies the nutrients required for the growth of the ectopic endometrium but also may be an important way for the transfer of endometrial cells from the normal intima to the myometrium. In terms of molecular biology, adenomyosis VEGF with its angiogenic activity at EMI is significantly enhanced but does not change with the proliferation and secretion phase; VEGF not only accelerates the uterine endometrial gland invasion but also promotes ectopic endothelial cell proliferation. All the above findings support the theory of increased angiogenesis as the pathogenesis of adenomyosis.

2.7   High Estrogen and High Prolactin Theory

Patients with endometriosis have abnormal hypothalamic-pituitary-ovarian axis function and often have corpus luteum dysfunction. Both adenomyosis and endometriosis are estrogen-dependent diseases. Anti-estrogen drugs are used to treat endometriosis as well as adenomyosis. Obviously, androgen is the root cause of adenomyosis.

Aromatase, also called estrogen synthetase or estrogen synthase, is an enzyme responsible for a key step in the biosynthesis of estrogens. Patients with adenomyosis have high expression of aromatase in the endometrium, but in the endometrium of women without adenomyosis, its expression is difficult to be detected. In addition to aromatase, the activity of 17β-hydroxysteroid dehydrogenase type 2 that decomposes estrogen decreases, which ultimately leads to a high-estrogen environment in adenomyosis. After the estrogen combines with the corticotropin-releasing hormone and urocortin in the adenomyosis, these hormones stimulate cyclooxygenase and its isoenzyme COX-2, to make an increase in PGE2. Both COX-2 and PGE2 are powerful inducers of aromatase activity and exert a positive feedback mechanism to aggravate dysmenorrhea. It is suggested that estrogen can indirectly promote uterine contraction and coordinate with oxytocin to regulate uterine contractility. Therefore the locally increased estrogen in adenomyosis can regulate uterine contractility, resulting in abnormal contractions and increased peristalsis of the sub-endometrial myometrium. That is why the use of aromatase inhibitors to treat adenomyosis can reduce the uterine volume of adenomyosis and dysmenorrhea. It has the same effect as gestrinone. This finding supports the increase of estrogen levels in patients with adenomyosis; especially the local high estrogen environment is the main cause of adenomyosis [45].

In addition to estrogen, hyperprolactinemia can also directly induce adenomyosis. Prolactin can promote the binding of estrogen to its receptors and increase the effective biological activity of estrogen.

2.8   Immune Factors

Recent studies have found that the onset of adenomyosis may be related to abnormalities in humoral immunity, cellular immunity, and cytokines [45, 46]. In terms of humoral immunity, patients with adenomyosis may have abnormalities in immunoglobulin and complement. Abnormal cellular immunity of adenomyosis mainly includes natural killer cell reduction, macrophage increase, and helper T cell 1/ helper T cell 2 (Th1/Th2) cell imbalance. The reduction of the killing capacity of natural killer cells is beneficial to the implantation of endometrial cells in the myometrium. After activation, macrophages can secrete a variety of inflammatory factors, such as interleukin (IL) -1β and TNF-α, and increase the oxidation reaction, resulting in increased oxygen consumption, resulting in oxidative stress, which in turn has a toxic effect on the embryo, affecting embryo implantation, and reduce the pregnancy rate. After treatment with GnRHa, the number of macrophage infiltration in the endometrium and uterine myometrium of patients with adenomyosis was significantly reduced and accompanied by a significant reduction of monocyte chemoattractant protein, (MCP -1), thereby increasing the clinical pregnancy rate of patients with adenomyosis, which may explain the immunological mechanism of adenomyosis with infertility [47].

2.9   Genes and Genetic Factors

Genetic factors may be involved in the occurrence of adenomyosis, but this process requires the joint action of external factors. At present, no single gene has been found that directly leads to the formation of adenomyosis. Studies have shown that related gene changes may be involved in the occurrence and development of adenomyosis, which is mainly achieved through apoptosis regulation, proliferation regulation, and mutation and inactivation of tumor suppressor genes [48, 49]. In adenomyosis lesions, the apoptosis control gene Bcl-2 shows continuous high expression without periodic changes, and the local ectopic endometrial tissue and the influence of the internal environment can up-regulate its expression. The existence of Bcl-2 protein prevents ectopic endometrial cells of the adenomyosis from expressing and triggering cell surface receptors related to apoptosis, which reduces apoptosis and increases cell proliferation. It, in turn, promotes the occurrence and development of adenomyosis. At the same time, the high expression of survivin protein in the ectopic endometrial gland of adenomyosis significantly enhances the anti-apoptosis ability of ectopic endometrial cells. It also slows down apoptosis, thereby prolonging the survival time of endometrial cells invading the myometrium. Therefore, the high level of survivin protein may also be one of the causes of adenomyosis. In the uterine endometrium and ectopic endometrium of adenomyosis patients, the expression intensity of Fas/FasL is significantly weakened, and the imbalance causes ectopic endometrial cells to survive and escape the attacks from the body's immune system, which is an important mechanism for the pathogenesis of adenomyosis [50]. Adenomyosis patients have overexpression of many other genes closely related to cell proliferation, which promotes the growth of the intima, which leads to the occurrence and development of adenomyosis. These related genes mainly include proliferating cell nuclear antigen, proto-oncogene c-myc, proto-oncogene TrkB, and pituitary tumor transformation genes. The expression of these genes can promote cell proliferation, regulate the cell cycle, inhibit cell secretion, regulate apoptosis, promote cell migration, ectopic attachment, angiogenesis, and invasion, and ultimately promote the occurrence of adenomyosis [51]. Also, the inactivation of tumor suppressor genes and the occurrence of adenomyosis are closely related to the occurrence and development of adenomyosis [49].

In addition to epigenetic involvement in the pathogenesis of adenomyosis, a variety of oncogenes or tumor suppressor genes, metabolic genes, and cell signal regulation genes (or factors) have been found in recent years that may be related to the onset of adenomyosis. Because these oncogenes or metabolic genes can proliferate and invade, adenomyosis with these genes also has the characteristics of invasion and metastasis; therefore, most of the current researches use the discovered oncogenes to study adenomyosis.

In endometriosis, galectin-33 can up-regulate the expression of NGF. High expression of galectin-33 was also present in adenomyosis, and the induced high expression of NGF can promote ectopic endometrial proliferation and is related to the patient's pain. Because endometriosis has the biological behavior characteristics of malignant tumors, it is believed that some malignant biological behavior characteristics of endometriosis also exist in adenomyosis. For example, the onset of endometriosis involves mitogen-activated protein kinase (MAPK), Akt/protein kinase B (PKB), NF-κB, and phosphatidylinositol 3-kinase (Phosphatidylinositol3-kinase, PI3K), and other cell signaling pathways [52]. The pathogenesis of adenomyosis also involves these cell signaling pathways. However, patients with endometriosis have a family aggregation phenomenon, and adenomyosis is not yet clear whether this phenomenon exists. Therefore, the genetic research involving adenomyosis still needs much work.

2.10   Inflammation or Infection Factors

Most researchers have recognized the role of inflammation in the pathogenesis of endometriosis. Not surprisingly, many studies of ectopic endometrium and endometriosis showed a significant increase in IL-6 and other cytokines [53, 54]. Similarly, it is believed that inflammation or infection factors would also exist in adenomyosis. Therefore in patients with adenomyosis, whether it is serum or peritoneal fluid or endometrial tissue, abnormally elevated levels of IL-6 had been detected [55]. This finding showed that inflammation could be a causative factor of adenomyosis. The latest research also found that a variety of pathogenic microorganisms was detected in the vagina and cervical secretions of patients with adenomyosis, which was significantly higher than that of normal women [56]. This clinical finding, therefore, has a practical significance for the prevention and treatment of clinical adenomyosis.

2.11   Others

The incidence of adenomyosis has increased significantly in recent years. In addition to changes in people's lifestyles, environmental factors cannot be ignored. Stem cell receptors can be found in the endometrium of adenomyosis, especially at the junction of the endometrium and myometrium, namely JZ. Therefore, it is speculated that stem cells may also play a role in the pathogenesis of adenomyosis. Also, the bone marrow stem cell theory, biochemical theory, lymphatic dissemination, oxidative stress, and free radicals are considered to be involved in the pathogenesis of endometriosis. However, whether these phenomena or theories can be applied to the pathogenesis of adenomyosis still need much research to confirm.

In short, the pathogenesis of adenomyosis remains unclear. Although the above studies found that adenomyosis may be related to various factors, these factors do not act alone but a combination of various factors. Under the influence of various factors, such as uterine trauma, inflammation, or the patient's immune deficiency or possible inheritance, and migration and invasion capabilities of the endometrial cells, the endometrium then invades the myometrium, resulting in adenomyosis. It is believed that the pathogenesis of adenomyosis will be clarified and elucidated after more intensive researches in the future.

References

1. Graziano A, et al. Diagnostic findings in adenomyosis: a pictorial review on the major concerns. Eur Rev Med Pharmacol Sci. 2015;19(7):1146–54.
2. Tellum T, et al. Development of a clinical prediction model for diagnosing adenomyosis. Fertil Steril. 2018;110(5):957–964.e3.
3. Karamanidis D, et al. OC01: Transvaginal ultrasonography compared with magnetic resonance imaging for the diagnosis of adenomyosis. Ultrasound Obstet Gynecol. 2018;52(4):555.

4. Scoutt LM, et al. Junctional zone of the uterus: correlation of MR imaging and histologic examination of hysterectomy specimens. Radiology. 1991;179(2):403–7.
5. Agostinho L, et al. MRI for adenomyosis: a pictorial review. Insights Imaging. 2017;8(6):549–56.
6. Riggs JC, et al. Cesarean section as a risk factor for the development of adenomyosis uteri. J Reprod Med. 2014;59(1–2):20–4.
7. Leyendecker G, Wildt L. A new concept of endometriosis and adenomyosis: tissue injury and repair (TIAR). Horm Mol Biol Clin Invest. 2011;5(2):125–42.
8. Li T, Li Y-G, Pu D-M. Matrix metalloproteinase-2 and-9 expression correlated with angiogenesis in human adenomyosis. Gynecol Obstet Investig. 2006;62(4):229–35.
9. Xiao Y, et al. Expression of integrin β3 and osteopontin in the eutopic endometrium of adenomyosis during the implantation window. Eur J Obstet Gynecol Reprod Biol. 2013;170(2):419–22.
10. Hricak H, et al. Magnetic resonance imaging of the female pelvis: initial experience. Am J Roentgenol. 1983;141(6):1119–28.
11. Yifu S. There are some questions about uterine adenopathy. China Fam Plan Obstet Gynecol. 2018;10(1):3–6.
12. Leyendecker G, et al. Adenomyosis and endometriosis. Re-visiting their association and further insights into the mechanisms of auto-traumatisation. An MRI study. Arch Gynecol Obstet. 2015;291(4):917–32.
13. Shaked S, et al. Uterine peristalsis-induced stresses within the uterine wall may sprout adenomyosis. Biomech Model Mechanobiol. 2015;14(3):437–44.
14. Uduwela A, et al. Endometrial-myometrial interface: relationship to adenomyosis and changes in pregnancy. Obstet Gynecol Surv. 2000;55(6):390–400.
15. Liu Jingjing DH. Wangsha the expression and significance of nitric oxide in the smooth muscle cells in the endometrial-myoline junction region of uterine adenopathic patients. Chinese J Obstet Gynecol. 2013;48(007):504–7.
16. Kyo S, et al. Telomerase activity in gynecological tumors. Clin Cancer Res. 1996;2(12):2023–8.
17. Xue Q, Zhou Y, Liu Y. Expression of ki67 and CA_ (125) in Adenomyosis. J Pract Obstet Gynecol. 2003;5
18. Deng Y, Chunlan H, Xiaoling L. Expression of Survivin in Adenomyosis and its relationship with Bcl-2 and Bax protein. J Med Res. 2006;6
19. Xiao Y, et al. Expression of integrin beta3 and osteopontin in endometrium of patients with adenomyosis. Zhonghua Fu Chan Ke Za Zhi. 2009;44(5):354–8.
20. Polyak K, Weinberg RA. Transitions between epithelial and mesenchymal states: acquisition of malignant and stem cell traits. Nat Rev Cancer. 2009;9(4):265–73.
21. Acloque H, et al. Epithelial-mesenchymal transitions: the importance of changing cell state in development and disease. J Clin Invest. 2009;119(6):1438–49.
22. An M, et al. Interaction of macrophages and endometrial cells induces epithelial–mesenchymal transition-like processes in adenomyosis. Biol Reprod. 2017;96(1):46–57.
23. Khan KN, et al. Involvement of hepatocyte growth factor-induced epithelial-mesenchymal transition in human adenomyosis. Biol Reprod. 2015;92(2):35. 1-11
24. Oh SJ, et al. β-Catenin activation contributes to the pathogenesis of adenomyosis through epithelial–mesenchymal transition. J Pathol. 2013;231(2):210–22.
25. Chen YJ, et al. Oestrogen-induced epithelial–mesenchymal transition of endometrial epithelial cells contributes to the development of adenomyosis. J Pathol. 2010;222(3):261–70.
26. Sobel V, Zhu Y-S, Imperato-McGinley J. Fetal hormones and sexual differentiation. Obstet Gynecol Clin. 2004;31(4):837–56.
27. Spencer TE, et al. Comparative developmental biology of the mammalian uterus. Curr Top Dev Biol. 2005;68:85–122.
28. Donnez J, et al. Stereometric evaluation of peritoneal endometriosis and endometriotic nodules of the rectovaginal septum. Hum Reprod. 1996;11(1):224–8.

29. Enatsu A, et al. Adenomyosis in a patient with the Rokitansky-Kuster-Hauser syndrome. Fertil Steril. 2000;73(4):862–3.
30. Gargett CE. Uterine stem cells: what is the evidence? Hum Reprod Update. 2007;13(1):87–101.
31. Chan RW, Schwab KE, Gargett CE. Clonogenicity of human endometrial epithelial and stromal cells. Biol Reprod. 2004;70(6):1738–50.
32. Kato K. Stem cells in human normal endometrium and endometrial cancer cells: characterization of side population cells. Kaohsiung J Med Sci. 2012;28(2):63–71.
33. Long Wenjie GL, Fudi L, Xin S, Hui L. Stem cells and their relationship with adenomyosis*. Prog Mod Biomed. 2017;17(2):393–5.
34. Taylor HS. Endometrial cells derived from donor stem cells in bone marrow transplant recipients. JAMA. 2004;292(1):81–5.
35. Zhang W-B, et al. A study in vitro on differentiation of bone marrow mesenchymal stem cells into endometrial epithelial cells in mice. Eur J Obstet Gynecol Reprod Biol. 2012;160(2):185–90.
36. Morelli SS, Rameshwar P, Goldsmith LT. Experimental evidence for bone marrow as a source of nonhematopoietic endometrial stromal and epithelial compartment cells in a murine model. Biol Reprod. 2013;89(1):1–7.
37. Du H, Naqvi H, Taylor HS. Ischemia/reperfusion injury promotes and granulocyte-colony stimulating factor inhibits migration of bone marrow-derived stem cells to endometrium. Stem Cells Dev. 2012;21(18):3324–31.
38. Ibrahim MG, et al. Ultramicro-trauma in the endometrial-myometrial junctional zone and pale cell migration in adenomyosis. Fertil Steril. 2015;104(6):1475–1483.e3.
39. Zhang Yumin ZS. The study of pale cells and adenomyosis. Chin J Obstet Gynecol. 2018;1:39.
40. Zhang X, et al. Endometrial nerve fibers in women with endometriosis, adenomyosis, and uterine fibroids. Fertil Steril. 2009;92(5):1799–801.
41. Choi YS, et al. Effects of LNG-IUS on nerve growth factor and its receptors expression in patients with adenomyosis. Growth Factors. 2010;28(6):452–60.
42. Ota H, Tanaka T. Stromal vascularization in the endometrium during adenomyosis. Microsc Res Tech. 2003;60(4):445–9.
43. Mu Y, et al. Serum levels of vascular endothelial growth factor and cancer antigen 125 are related to the prognosis of adenomyosis patients after interventional therapy. Int J Clin Exp Med. 2015;8(6):9549.
44. Liu X, et al. Corroborating evidence for platelet-induced epithelial-mesenchymal transition and fibroblast-to-myofibroblast transdifferentiation in the development of adenomyosis. Hum Reprod. 2016;31(4):734–49.
45. Garcia L, Isaacson K. Adenomyosis: review of the literature. J Minim Invasive Gynecol. 2011;18(4):428–37.
46. Ota H, et al. Is adenomyosis an immune disease? Hum Reprod Update. 1998;4(4):360–7.
47. Garavaglia E, et al. Adenomyosis and its impact on women fertility. Iran J Reprod Med. 2015;13(6):327.
48. Vannuccini S, et al. Pathogenesis of adenomyosis: an update on molecular mechanisms. Reprod Biomed Online. 2017;35(5):592–601.
49. Liu Y, et al. Down-regulation of tumor suppressor PDCD4 expression in endometrium of adenomyosis patients. Current Res Transl Med. 2016;64(3):123–8.
50. Ye F, Zhang J, Qin J-q. Expression and significance of COX-2 and VEGF in adenomyosis. J Harbin Med Univ. 2006;3
51. Huang Y, et al. Expression of tyrosine kinase receptor B in eutopic endometrium of women with adenomyosis. Arch Gynecol Obstet. 2011;283(4):775–80.

52. Cakmak H, et al. Immune-endocrine interactions in endometriosis. Front Biosci (Elite Ed). 2009;1(2):429–43.
53. Keenan JA, et al. Interferon-gamma (IFN-γ) and Interleukin-6 (IL-6) in peritoneal fluid and macrophage-conditioned Media of Women with Endometriosis. Am J Reprod Immunol. 1994;32(3):180–3.
54. Bergqvist A, et al. Interleukin 1β, interleukin-6, and tumor necrosis factor-α in endometriotic tissue and in endometrium. Fertil Steril. 2001;75(3):489–95.
55. Yang JH, et al. Increased interleukin-6 messenger RNA expression in macrophage-cocultured endometrial stromal cells in adenomyosis. Am J Reprod Immunol. 2006;55(3):181–7.
56. Chen C, et al. The microbiota continuum along the female reproductive tract and its relation to uterine-related diseases. Nat Commun. 2017;8(1):1–11.

The Pathology of Adenomyosis

3

Fang Xiao and Min Xue

Adenomyosis is a benign penetration of the endometrium into the muscle layer of the uterus. Characteristically, there are endometrial glands and interstitial cell islands in the myometrium, accompanied by hyperplasia and hypertrophy of the surrounding smooth muscle tissue. Cullen in 1908 [1] studied 73 consecutive cases of adenomyosis; 56 cases were found to be connected to the endometrium, so it is generally accepted that adenomyosis comes from the endometrial glands and stroma. Although trauma to the endometrium lining is conducive to the invasion of the glands into the myometrium, to form the adenomyosis, it is difficult to explain why adenomyosis occurs in women who have not had uterine surgery, such as uterine curetting or myomectomy. The reason why the endometrial glands invade the myometrium remains unclear; various theories of its pathogenesis have been mentioned in the previous chapter.

Mai et al. 1997 [2] suggested that isolated and multipotent pericytes exist in the vicinity of blood vessels or lymphatic vessels in the myometrium; they proliferate and fuse with the surrounding tissue then form the adenomyosis. Adenomyosis is different from endometriosis, in which the endometriosis appears outside of the myometrium. However, endometriosis can invade the uterus from the pelvis and accumulate behind the serosa and invade into the outer muscular layer of the uterine wall. Endometriosis will not be connected to the uterine endometrium nor will it be accompanied by hyperplasia and hypertrophy of the muscle tissue.

Adenomyosis shows no sharp boundary between the endometrium and the myometrium, whereas the boundary demonstrates irregular finger-like protrusions. When the glands and stroma of the endometrium have penetrated the muscle layer excessively, it is called adenomyosis. Due to a lack of clear definition, the pathological diagnosis of adenomyosis is somewhat arbitrary. The true incidence of

F. Xiao (✉) · M. Xue
Department of Gynecology and Obstetrics, Third Xiangya Hospital of Central South University, Changsha, Hunan, China

adenomyosis is difficult to determine. The reported incidence is 1–70%, which is very different. This vast difference could be due to the different histopathological criteria of diagnosis, the different indications of uterine surgery, the locations, and the number of the tissue biopsies taken. Among them, the main problem is the differences in the pathological diagnostic criteria. Also, the difference in the incidence of adenomyosis may be related to different hospital practices.

3.1 Macroscopic Appearance of Adenomyosis

If the adenomyosis is mild, the uterus can be normal in size, and in patients with obvious clinical symptoms, the uterus is often enlarged (Fig. 3.1). Mostly the increase in the size of the uterus is caused by the hypertrophy of the uterine smooth muscle cells that accompanies the invasion of the endometrium. Very few are caused by the endometrial cells itself. There are two types of adenomyosis lesions: diffused and localized.

1. Diffused type: Due to the adenomyosis, the uterus is diffusely, uniformly, and spherically enlarged. Sometimes, a huge uterus is caused by adenomyosis associated with uterine fibroids. Macroscopically the adenomyosis shows that the involved muscular layer is thickened and hardened, generally, about 2–4 cm and the thickness can reach up to 6–7 cm, or even thicker, and the wall thickening is more common in the posterior uterine wall. Posterior wall adenomyosis accounts for more than half of the adenomyosis. Thick fibromuscular bands can be seen in the myometrium in the affected area, showing a swirling and braided structure, but unlike fibroids, no nodules are formed. There is no clear boundary between the adenomyosis and the surrounding myometrial tissue, and there is no pseudo-capsule. There are small dark-red or purple-blue cracks between the hypertro-phic muscle bundles, which can be very small like a needle tip, or it can expand up to several millimeters to form a microcapsule cavity, which is filled with

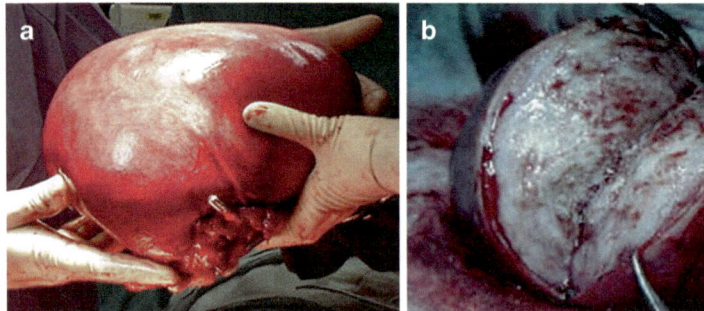

Fig. 3.1 Gross appearance of an enlarged uterus with adenomyosis and small fibroids. (**a**) A large uterus with adenomyosis removed by hysterectomy (**b**) Cut surface of the uterus with adenomyosis showed diffused adenomyosis lesions

bluish or dark-red old blood. Sometimes there is no bleeding inside the lesion, which becomes a transparent and soft sponge-like area, which mixes between the hypertrophic muscle bundles.

2. Localized type: Adenomyosis can grow in a localized form in the myometrium to form nodules or clumps, similar to intramural fibroids of the uterus, and it is also known as "adenomyoma." The uterus will appear irregular and nodular in shape. The normal uterine muscle tissue at the lesion is hard and tough, and it feels nodular when touched. Macroscopically on the cut surface of the uterus, there are single or multiple nodules in the muscular layer. This nodule is like a leiomyoma in the uterine myometrium, but it does not have a pseudocapsule and cannot be completely peeled off during the surgery. Occasionally, pedicled adenomyoma protruded into the uterine cavity, resembling a submucosal fibroid. The cut surfaces of adenomyosis nodules show small cavities with blood or translucent sponge-like areas. Sometimes localized adenomyoma affects the uterine cornua, presenting as unilateral or double horns of a uterus, usually about 1 cm in diameter; the cut surface shows areas of muscular hyperplasia, with small bleeding cavities or mixed with translucent sponge-like areas. Sometimes a nodule arising from salpingitis appears similar to adenomyoma, but they are different diseases [3]. The nodule is salpingitis isthmica nodosa, which appears like an adenomatous structure at the isthmus of the fallopian tube; it may block the fallopian tube and cause infertility.

In rare cases, adenomyosis forms a large cyst cavity in the muscular layer, and its clinical symptoms are like ovarian cysts. Sometimes rupture of the cyst cavity of adenomyosis can cause internal bleeding. It is rare for endometriosis to occur in leiomyoma to form an adenomyoma. However, even it is rare, this kind of lesion, like fibroids, has a pseudocapsule, and the whole lesion can be peeled off completely.

3.2   Microscopic Appearance of Adenomyosis

Microscopic examination of adenomyosis [4] showed sheet or island-like endometrial tissues with uneven density, unequal size, and different positions in the uterine myometrium. The number of endometrial glands varies from only one to four or five or even more. The diagnosis of typical adenomyosis is not difficult. Occasionally, the number of glands in the lesion of adenomyosis is sparse or even not obvious or none at all. Only islands of interstitial cells are seen scattered in the muscle layer, which can be similar to the low-grade endometrial stromal sarcoma. If accompanied by the expansion of stromal veins, it is more like a low-grade endometrial stromal sarcoma. However, the stromal cells in adenomyosis without glands show a single, uniform nucleus, no atypical nucleus, and no active mitosis with surrounding hypertrophic smooth muscle tissue. In other parts of the adenomyosis lesions, some typical glandular and interstitial components of adenomyosis can still be seen, which can be distinguished from the low-grade endometrial stromal sarcoma. This scarcity of glands in the lesion is occasionally seen in post-menopausal adenomyosis, because the glands may shrink like endometrial atrophy after menopause.

The morphological changes in the lesions of adenomyosis can be similar to the eutopic endometrium. The most common changes are similar to that of immature glands and stroma in the basal layer of the endometrium. This endometrium responds only to estrogen but not to progesterone. When the uterine endometrium has been changed to the secretory phase of the cycle, the glands and stroma in the adenomyosis are still in the proliferative phase, and the stromal cells will not show decidual changes. Sometimes glandular cells in adenomyosis can undergo meta-plastic changes, and squamous metaplasia can occur. When estrogen imbalance occurs, the endometrial glands of adenomyosis can also show various forms of endometrial hyperplasia. The appearances show increased number of glands, vary-ing sizes of gland cavity, cystic or glandular, back-to-back, glandular irregularity, and glandular epithelial cell hyperplasia forming protrusions into the gland cavity; in severe cases, it may be accompanied by atypical glandular epithelial changes, with enlargement of cell nuclei, different sizes and shapes, increased chromatin and active mitosis presenting as simple endometrial hyperplasia, complex hyperplasia, and atypical hyperplasia.

In a few cases, the ectopic endometrium of adenomyosis may have different degrees of functional activities. Occasionally, the ectopic endometrium exhibits the same periodic and functional response as the normal endometrium, manifesting as proliferative, secretory, and stromal cell decidualization as in the menstrual cycle. However, during the secretory phase, the ectopic endometrium of adenomyosis often manifests as various forms: uneven secretory changes, secretory in some areas, and proliferative phase in other areas; even in the same secretory phase, some glands secrete better and some poorer, and they are often in either early, middle, or late secretory phases which cannot be distinguished. In pregnancy, the ectopic endo-metrial glands of adenomyosis show a highly secretory state; the interstitial cells become large with the cytoplasm being rich, bright, and interleaved, showing the characteristics of decidual cells.

3.3   Malignant Transformation of Adenomyosis

Malignant transformation of adenomyosis is rare and seldom reported. Its scarcity may be related to the following factors. First, early diagnosis of malignant transfor-mation of adenomyosis is difficult. The specific clinical symptoms of malignant transformation of adenomyosis are mostly unintentionally found in the surgical and pathological examination of the excised specimen. Secondly, the most important point in the diagnostic criteria for malignant transformation of adenomyosis is to be able to determine the origin of malignant lesions in the epithelial or interstitial areas of adenomyosis. It requires the transitional areas of malignant lesions and adeno-myosis to be seen in the pathological sections. When malignant adenomyosis changes are at its advanced stage, the malignant tissue invades the actual uterine endometrium and even replaces it completely. It makes it difficult to judge the true origin of the malignancy. Therefore, there could be some cases being diagnosed as endometrial cancer with adenomyosis. Because there is no clear diagnostic basis of its origin, it is often classified as the uterine endometrial cancer.

Whether reported cases of malignant transformation of adenomyosis are all true, adenocarcinoma is still controversial. In a study of 50 cases of adenomyosis, Colman et al. 1959 [5] found 7 cases of adenomyosis with abnormal changes in the endometrial glandular epithelium, only 1 case of adenocarcinoma in situ, 2 cases of hyperplasia, and 4 cases of cancers in both the adenomyosis and uterine endometrium. It suggested that abnormal changes in the ectopic endometrium of the adenomyosis are relatively common. Some of the reported malignant adenomyosis may be a type of abnormal hyperplastic changes in adenomyosis, rather than true adenocarcinoma. According to the strict criteria used by Sampson 1925 [6] to diagnose malignant transformation of endometriosis, the proposed criteria are: (a) There are no malignant lesions in the uterine endometrium and pelvic area. (b) Cancer must be seen arising from the glandular epithelium of adenomyosis, and it must have a transition or continuous area between the benign endometrial glands and cancerous glands, rather than invading or metastasizing from other parts. (c) The endometrial stroma must be seen around the cancerous lesion to support the evidence of adenomyosis. Fortunately, patients with malignant transformation of adenomyosis have an excellent prognosis after surgery.

It is often difficult to distinguish between endometrial adenocarcinoma involving adenomyosis or primary adenomyosis cancer from its carcinogenesis. Therefore, at this time, the uterine endometrium must be thoroughly and carefully checked to determine whether there is cancer in the endometrium. After excluding endometrial adenocarcinoma involving adenomyosis, the malignant transformation of adenomyosis can be diagnosed. According to the current research, the three conditions, malignant transformation of adenomyosis, endometrial adenocarcinoma involving adenomyosis, and endometrial adenocarcinoma invades the myometrium, should have a strict difference in the diagnostic concept. The pathology should make a clear diagnosis of the three conditions to avoid inappropriate treatment of the patients.

3.4   Pathological Changes After Focused Ultrasound Treatment

Because of the various severe symptoms of adenomyosis, there are many medical and surgical treatments. The only effective treatment proven by evidence-based medicine is hysterectomy. This traditional treatment not only completely leads to a total loss of reproductive function, but it also causes pelvic floor dysfunction, perimenopausal symptoms, and premature ovarian failure. There are other related psychiatric syndromes, including postpartum depression, premenstrual syndrome (PMS), post-hysterectomy depression, and involutional melancholia. These syndromes will lead to a loss of confidence and a decline in the quality of life [7]. Also, due to the misunderstanding of the sexual functions of the uterus and the husband's misconception about the loss of the uterus, it may cause the loss of libido and the quality of sexual life of the couple, thus affecting family stability and social harmony. Therefore, the high-intensity focused ultrasound (HIFU), uterine artery embolization, and other conservative uterus-preserving surgeries are often used to manage this condition.

Although HIFU ablation for adenomyosis to be discussed in this book has good safety and effectiveness in the treatment of adenomyosis from a basic and clinical perspective, there are, however, only a few reports on the pathological changes related to adenomyosis after these treatments.

Yang et al. 2003 [8] conducted an in vivo HIFU treatment for a localized adenomyoma before a hysterectomy procedure. After HIFU treatment, the tissues in the irradiated area were grayish-white, dry, and regular, with a hard texture. The staining with 2,3,5-triphenyltetrazolium chloride (TTC) showed that the tissues in the sonication area were not stained, presented as grayish-white, regular evenly red-stained areas. The boundary between the two was clear.

After HIFU treatment, the adenomyosis tissues showed different degrees of coagulative necrosis, and the boundaries with the surrounding tissues were clear. The main manifestations were the destruction of glandular structures and the disappearance of cilia in glandular cells in the necrotic area. Glandular epithelial cells, interstitial cells, and smooth muscle cells had scattered nuclear shrinkage, nuclear rupture, enhanced cytoplasmic eosin staining, reduced nuclear volume, deeper chromosomes, and damage to the cell membrane, demonstrated by electron microscopy. Some early apoptotic cells also appeared in the vicinity. These cells showed mitochondrial swelling, vacuolar-like changes, cytoplasmic concentration, and formation of apoptotic bodies. The secretion of cytokines and proteins related to apoptosis increases and accelerates the occurrence of apoptosis. These are the pathological changes after HIFU ablation treatment for adenomyosis.

References

1. Cullen TS. Adenomyoma of the uterus. J Am Med Assoc. 1908;50(2):107–15.
2. Mai K, et al. Pathogenetic role of the stromal cells in endometriosis and adenomyosis. Histopathology. 1997;30(5):430–42.
3. Chawla N, et al. Salpingitis isthmica nodosa. Indian J Pathol Microbiol. 2009;52(3):434.
4. Zhang Bin LA-d, Xiangmei Z. Clinico-pathological analysis of 215 patients with adenomyosis. Fujian Med J. 2010;32(1):76–7.
5. Colman HI, Rosenthal AH. Carcinoma developing in areas of adenomyosis. Obstet Gynecol. 1959;14(3):342–8.
6. Sampson JA. Endometrial carcinoma of the ovary, arising in endometrial tissue in that organ. Arch Surg. 1925;10(1):1–72.
7. Gitlin MJ, Pasnau RO. Psychiatric syndromes linked to reproductive function in women: a review of current knowledge. Am J Psychiatry. 1989;146(11):1413–22.
8. Yang Zhu CY, Lina H, Zhixuan W (2003) The preliminary study of pathological changes of adenomyosis in human body after high-intensity focused ultrasound therapy clinical ultrasound Medicine

The Clinical Features and Diagnosis of Adenomyosis

4

Yi Dai and Jinhua Leng

As early as 1920, Cullen [1] described adenomyosis as "endometriosis with predominantly presence of fibromuscular tissue," and in 1921 Sampson [2] distinguished three types of adenomyosis. However, adenomyosis remained little known in the later decades and written only as an appendix in books on endometriosis, not knowing that adenomyosis has a great adverse impact on women's health. For a long time, adenomyosis could only be diagnosed on histological specimens after hysterectomy in reproductive age women with heavy menstrual bleeding or pelvic pain [3]. Therefore the incidence rate in retrospective studies was seriously underestimated, and the prevalence rate varies due to the criteria used. Over the last 10 years, adenomyosis has become a condition diagnosed in young reproductive age women [4] because of the recent advancements in imaging techniques. Despite the new diagnostic tools, the awareness of the disease is still poor among the doctors with consensus on definition, and classification is still lacking [5]. Furthermore, adenomyosis is often associated with other gynecological conditions, such as endometriosis and fibroids. This chapter will discuss the clinical features and diagnosis of adenomyosis.

The diagnosis of adenomyosis should first be based on the patient's history, clinical symptoms, and signs. Imaging examination is an important basis for the diagnosis of adenomyosis, but the gold standard for the diagnosis is still pathological diagnosis.

Y. Dai · J. Leng (✉)
Department of Obstetrics and Gynecology, Peking Union Medical College Hospital, Beijing, China

© The Author(s), under exclusive license to Springer Nature Singapore Pte Ltd. 2021
M. Xue et al. (eds.), *Adenomyosis*, https://doi.org/10.1007/978-981-33-4095-4_4

4.1 Pathology Diagnosis

The diagnosis of adenomyosis has always been from the histological examination of hysterectomy specimens [6, 7] in the past. The disease is commonly confirmed histologically by the presence of endometrial glands and stroma located deep within the myometrium, associated with smooth muscle hyperplasia [8] (Fig. 4.1). It is the invasion of the myometrium by basal glands and stroma with the destruction of normal myometrium architecture [7, 9]. Nevertheless, the incidence of adenomyosis can vary widely, depending on the diagnostic criteria among different pathologists, because there are no uniform criteria regarding the depth of invasion and number of foci to make a diagnosis, especially when the disease is not diffuse. For example, to make a diagnosis of adenomyosis, an invasion of more than one-third thickness of the myometrium is used as a criterion, whereas in others, a myometrial invasion >4 mm is diagnostic [10–12].

Histologically, adenomyosis is defined as focal when a nodular area of the endometrial glands and stroma are surrounded by normal myometrium. This focal lesion can present either as a muscular or cystic lesion. On the other hand, in diffuse adenomyosis, endometrial glands and stroma are recognized throughout the myometrium of the uterus. Diffuse adenomyosis is not well circumscribed and can involve either the posterior and/or anterior uterine wall partially or wholly, resulting in asymmetric enlargement of the uterus.

4.2 The Clinical Diagnosis

Adenomyosis affects the physical and mental health of patients. But only a small group of women undergo non-conservative surgical treatments for adenomyosis, because the introduction of new medications has allowed clinicians to treat the disease conservatively. Patients need early diagnosis of adenomyosis, so that early treatment and intervention can ensure her a better quality of life and reproductive outcomes. Many experts agree that adenomyosis requires a lifelong management plan, including pain, bleeding control, fertility support, and pregnancy outcome.

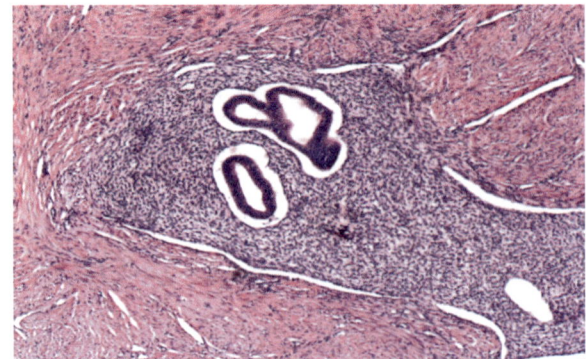

Fig. 4.1 Hematoxylin and eosin staining of adenomyosis (40 X). It shows a nodular area of the endometrial glands and stroma surrounded by a normal myometrium

Thus, a realistic treatment background cannot be established only from histopathology, which is often unavailable. Therefore the patient's history, clinical symptoms, and signs together with imaging examination are important for the diagnosis of adenomyosis.

4.3   History

4.3.1   Age

It had been reported that 70–80% of women undergoing hysterectomy for adenomyosis are in their fourth and fifth decade of life [13–15]. However, newer studies suggest that the disease may cause dysmenorrhea and chronic pelvic pain in adolescents and women of younger reproductive age by using MRI criteria for diagnosis [16, 17]. The age at their clinical presentation may be much earlier, and it may be a different clinical phenotype compared to adenomyosis of late onset.

4.3.2   Multiparity

Among women with adenomyosis, many are multiparous [3, 15, 18, 19]. As early as 1995, Vercellini et al. [20] reported in the Milan epidemiological study on adenomyosis that the frequency of adenomyosis was directly associated with the number of births and tended to be higher with spontaneous and induced abortions. The odds ratio of adenomyosis in women with one and more than two births was 1.3 and 1.5, respectively, compared with nulliparous women ($P < 0.05$). But in their study, there was no relationship between the risk of adenomyosis and age during surgery, age at menarche, indication for surgery, menopausal status at intervention, and the presence of endometriosis. In a cross-sectional study conducted on 707 consecutive women who underwent hysterectomy between 1993 and 1994 [21], the incidence of adenomyosis was higher in parous women, in comparison with nulliparae; the odds ratios of adenomyosis were 1.8 (95% CI 0.9–3.4) and 3.1 (95% CI 1.7–5.5), respectively, in women reporting one and more than two births ($P < 0.01$).

Pregnancy might facilitate the formation of adenomyosis due to the invasive nature of the trophoblast extending into the myometrial fibers, thus allowing ectopic endometrial foci from the endometrial-myometrium junctional zone to be included in the myometrium [18, 19]. Besides, adenomyosis has high-level estrogen receptors; thus, pregnancy with its hormonal milieu may favor the development of islands of ectopic endometrium [13].

4.3.3   History of Uterine Surgery

The history of operations involving the uterine cavity may be one of the risk factors of adenomyosis, even though there are still controversies. The assumption that surgical disruptions of the endometrial-myometrial border could result in endometrial glands invading the myometrial layer, with increasing risk of adenomyosis formation [14, 22]. In a cohort study of 1850 women with hysterectomy in over 4 years, Curtis et al. 2002 [23] analyzed the surgical disruption of the endometrial-myometrial junctional zone by sharp curettage as a risk factor for adenomyosis. For women who had a history of suction evacuation for termination of pregnancy, those with more than three abortions had an increased risk of adenomyosis of 5.9 (95% CI 1.5–23.3), and the risk increased with the number of abortions. Repeated sharp curettage during early pregnancy at the time of abortion may greatly increase the risk of adenomyosis by disrupting the endometrial-myometrial border and facilitating implantation, embedding, and survival of endometrium within the myometrial wall. Based on the understanding of wound healing, the endometrial-myometrial interface disruption (EMID) is proposed to cause adenomyosis resulting from iatrogenic trauma to endometrial myometrial interface (EMI) [24]. The EMID hypothesis includes many mechanisms, as presented in Fig. 4.2, i.e., hypoxia at the wounding site, platelet aggregation, angiogenesis, that enhanced survival of endometrial cells dispersed and displaced due to iatrogenic operations. This EMID hypothesis predicts that the risk of adenomyosis can be reduced if certain perioperative interventions are performed.

Interestingly, in the non-pregnant status, sharp curettage might not increase the risk. Panganamamula et al. studied 412 adenomyosis in 873 women (47%) who underwent hysterectomy for benign conditions within 8 years [22]. When individual types of surgery were analyzed separately, there were no significant differences between women with and without adenomyosis relating to previous cesarean delivery, myomectomy, endometrial ablation, dilatation and evacuation. However, after pooling all procedures, the history of any prior uterine surgery significantly increased the risk of adenomyosis (49% versus 41%; OR 1.37, 95% CI 1.05–1.79).

On the other hand, some studies reported no increased cesarean section or any other uterine surgical procedure in women with adenomyosis [3, 25, 26]. Therefore, it is still controversial that uterine surgery is a risk factor for adenomyosis. Moreover, the majority of the studies were conducted 10 years ago; the results from any new studies may well be different because of the advance in imaging technology and classification of adenomyosis.

4.3.4   Smoking

There are different views on the relationship between smoking and adenomyosis. Parazzini et al. 1997 [27] reported that smokers were less likely to have adenomyosis in comparison with women who never smoked. Adenomyosis is an estrogen-dependent lesion [8, 9, 28], and decreased serum levels of estrogen have been reported in smokers [29, 30]. Therefore this finding might explain the correlation. On the other hand, two studies reported a higher rate of women smokers with adenomyosis than in controls [3, 31]. Thus, we need further investigations to study the association between adenomyosis and smoking.

4.4   Symptoms

The clinical presentation and symptoms of adenomyosis are not discussed in detail here, because they are in other chapters of this book. This chapter only addressed the relationship between clinical manifestations and clinical diagnosis.

4.4.1   Pain

Progressive dysmenorrhea is a typical clinical symptom of adenomyosis; the incidence of dysmenorrhea was reported between 50 and 93.4% [3, 4, 32]. Women with adenomyosis and fibroids had an odds ratio of 3.4 (95% CI 1.8–6.4) to experience dysmenorrhea than women with only fibroids [3]. Some researchers described a linear correlation between the extent of the adenomyosis and the severity of dysmenorrhea [4, 33]. The mechanism of dysmenorrhea and pelvic pain is likely due to an increase in prostaglandins and increased nerve fibers in the adenomyosis [34, 35]. The focal proliferation of small-diameter nerve fibers was observed at the margins of adenomyosis in some uteri [35]. Another mechanism of pain is due to uterine hyperperistalsis and the increased oxytocin receptors in patients with adenomyosis; these all contribute to the severity of dysmenorrhea [36].

4.4.2   Abnormal Uterine Bleeding

Abnormal uterine bleeding has been described with enlarged uterus due to diffuse adenomyosis. Not only is there increased menstrual loss [37] but also there is a statistically significant correlation between the extent of adenomyosis and the severity of abnormal uterine bleeding [38, 39]. The PALM-COEIN (polyp; adenomyosis; leiomyoma; malignancy and hyperplasia; coagulopathy; ovulatory dysfunction; endometrial; iatrogenic; and not yet classified, International Federation of Gynecology and Obstetrics) classification [40] includes adenomyosis as a specific entity of abnormal uterine bleeding in reproductive aged women, and it is strictly associated with heavy menstrual bleeding. In hysterectomy specimens of patients with abnormal uterine bleeding, the prevalence of adenomyosis was 34.3–49% [41, 42]. The abnormal vaginal bleeding can be due to an increased uterine volume, increased vascularization, abnormal uterine contractions, and increased production of estrogen and prostaglandins.

4.4.3   Infertility

Adenomyosis has an adverse effect on women's fertility. The mechanism mainly includes the dysfunction of the endometrial-myometrial junctional zone, the change of endometrial receptivity, the imbalance of estrogen receptor and progesterone receptor regulation, the abnormal level of oxygen free radicals in the uterine cavity, and the disorder of immune regulation. Adenomyosis also has adverse effects on the outcome of in vitro fertilization embryo transfer (IVF-ET) [43], such as the decrease of implantation rate, clinical pregnancy rate, continuous pregnancy rate, and live birth rate and the increase of abortion rate and adverse obstetric outcomes, such as premature delivery and premature rupture of membranes [43–45]. In two recent meta-analyses, adenomyosis was associated with a 30% decrease in the likelihood of pregnancy [43, 45]. By delaying pregnancy to a later reproductive age span, this group of women will be associated with greater risks of adenomyosis, requiring advice for fertility problems [38].

Patients with adenomyosis, in terms of clinical symptoms, have the following typical clinical presentations: ① progressive and gradually increasing dysmenorrhea; ② menorrhea (and/or prolonged menstruation); ③ infertility; ④ adverse pregnancy history, such as repeated abortion and premature delivery; ⑤ gynecological examination can often feel the increase of uterine uniformity, spherical shape, or localized nodule bulge, posterior position, and poor uterine motility. Then, the diagnosis of adenomyosis should be considered. However, it also should be reminded that some patients with adenomyosis are asymptomatic [46].

4.4.4 Imaging

MRI and transvaginal ultrasonography (TVUS) imaging technology have allowed clinicians to make a non-invasive diagnosis of adenomyosis in women suffering from dysmenorrhea, abnormal uterine bleeding, and infertility. The accuracy of the transvaginal ultrasound in the diagnosis of adenomyosis is high with a mean sensitivity of 72% (95% confidence interval [CI] 65–79%), specificity of 81% (95% CI 77–85%) and area under the curve (AUC) of 0.84 [5, 47]. However, its diagnostic performance could be biased by the experience of the examiner [5]. MRI has the advantage that it is not operator-dependent, and diagnosis is based on objective image findings. The sensitivity could reach 77% (95% CI 67–85%), specificity of 89% (95% CI 84–92%) [47, 48], and AUC of 0.92. Then MRI appears to be more accurate than transvaginal ultrasound and also has an excellent soft tissue differentiation with a clear identification of the junctional zone. However, MRI is more expensive than ultrasound. The technology progress of MRI not only greatly offers an early diagnosis of adenomyosis but also become the basis of clinical classification of adenomyosis. Among clinical types based on MRI, there are several representative classifications. Kishi et al. classified adenomyosis into four subtypes according to the localization of adenomyosis in the inner or outer myometrium, i.e., intrinsic, extrinsic, intramural, and indeterminate1 [49]. Grimbizis et al. 2014 [50] suggested a clinico-histological classification, identifying them as diffuse, focal, and cystic adenomyosis. More recently, Bazot and Daraï 2018 [51] proposed more complex subtypes of type A to K, according to MRI features. However, a shared classification system has not been developed yet, as further research is needed to better understand the physiopathology of adenomyosis, its onset and progression, and the interpretation of imaging signs according to the pathogenic theories [7].

4.4.5   Laboratory Test

CA125 is a well-known tumor marker of ovarian cancer. However, its levels may also be elevated in several relatively benign gynecological conditions, such as endometriosis and adenomyosis. Several studies have reported that elevated CA125 levels are associated with adenomyosis [52]. Besides, Kil et al. 2015 [53] reported that the differential diagnosis of adenomyosis and myoma could be based on a cut-off value if 19 U/mL for CA125 to provide improved diagnostic performance. They also suggested that serum CA125 testing can be performed during the initial screening of women with possible adenomyosis to differentiate it from myoma. However, the diagnostic accuracy of using CA125 testing alone is limited.

4.4.6   Hysteroscopy

Hysteroscopy, a diagnostic procedure, which allows the direct visualization of the uterine cavity, is also useful in the diagnosis of adenomyosis. It is the use of a rigid hysteroscope, via the transcervical route and distending medium to examine the endometrial cavity. The procedure is well-tolerated in an out-patient environment. El-Toukhy et al. 2016 [54] demonstrated that hysteroscopy found 26% of unsuspected uterine pathology in patients with recurrent implantation failure and normal ultrasound examination. Hysteroscopy can become a useful diagnostic method in the diagnosis of adenomyosis. It can allow the biopsy of the endometrial-myometrial junction zone under direct hysteroscopic vision. Because the field of vision is limited to the surface of the endometrium, and it is an invasive procedure by biopsy, hysteroscopy cannot often be used as a definitive diagnosis.

Hysteroscopic adenomyotic images can become obvious after a surgical subendometrial exploration during hysteroscopic resection (Fig. 4.2). The following hysteroscopic features may also indicate the diagnosis of adenomyosis: irregular endometrium, small openings between the surfaces; clear hyperplastic blood vessels; the "strawberry sign" of the endometrium; deep blue- or chocolate-colored cystic hemorrhage on the surface; and fibrocystic changes in the intrauterine focus. In adenomyosis, the abnormal distribution of endometrial blood vessels can be seen in both proliferative and secretory phases. This phenomenon can be enhanced and fully visible by reducing the inflation pressure of the distending medium, thus confirming the hypothesis of "dysfunction of endometrium in adenomyosis."

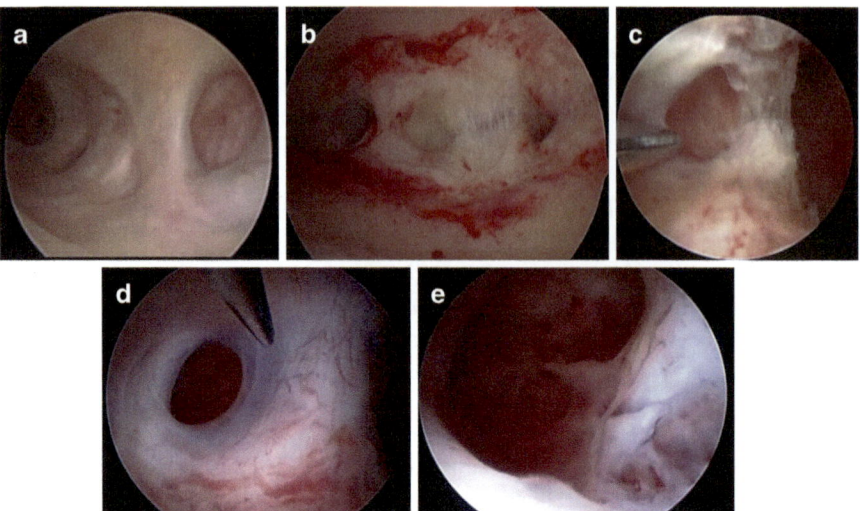

Fig. 4.2 (**a**) Visible endometrial defects; (**b**) after incision, different structures appear, showing adhesion and cystic opening; (**c**) after incision, an adenomyotic cystic opening becomes obvious; (**d**) other small cyst openings over the endometrial wall (**e**) a large cystic cavity is revealed after surgical incision of the cyst (reproduced with permission from Gordts's paper in Fertil Steril 2018)

4.5 Conclusion

Adenomyosis should be considered a chronic disease, which has an adverse impact on the physical and mental health of patients. Early and correct diagnosis, together with early intervention, can alleviate the suffering of patients, improve the quality of life, and improve the outcome of fertility. Despite controversies in the diagnosis and classifications of adenomyosis, the present information will serve as the direction of future research efforts.

References

1. Cullen TS. The distribution of adenomyomata containing uterine mucosa. Arch Surg. 1920;1:215–83.
2. Sampson J. Peritoneal endometriosis due to the menstrual dissemination of endometrial tissue into the peritoneal cavity. Am J Obstet Gynecol. 1927;14:422–69.
3. Taran FA, et al. Clinical characteristics indicating adenomyosis at the time of hysterectomy: a retrospective study in 291 patients. Arch Gynecol Obstet. 2012;285(6):1571–6.
4. Pinzauti S, et al. Transvaginal sonographic features of diffuse adenomyosis in 18-30-year-old nulligravid women without endometriosis: association with symptoms. Ultrasound Obstet Gynecol. 2015;46(6):730–6.
5. Van den Bosch T, Van Schoubroeck D. Ultrasound diagnosis of endometriosis and adenomyosis: state of the art. Best Pract Res Clin Obstet Gynaecol. 2018;51:16–24.
6. Abbott JA. Adenomyosis and abnormal uterine bleeding (AUB-A)-pathogenesis, diagnosis, and management. Best Pract Res Clin Obstet Gynaecol. 2017;40:68–81.

7. Vannuccini S, Petraglia F. Recent advances in understanding and managing adenomyosis. F1000Res. 2019;8:F1000 Faculty Rev-283.
8. Vannuccini S, et al. Pathogenesis of adenomyosis: an update on molecular mechanisms. Reprod Biomed Online. 2017;35(5):592–601.
9. Garcia-Solares J, et al. Pathogenesis of uterine adenomyosis: invagination or metaplasia? Fertil Steril. 2018;109(3):371–9.
10. Parra-Herran C, Howitt BE. Uterine Mesenchymal tumors: update on classification, staging, and molecular features. Surg Pathol Clin. 2019;12(2):363–96.
11. Zaloudek CJ, Soslow RA, Mesenchymal tumors of the uterus., in Blaustein's pathology of the female genital tract (6), Kurman RJ, . 2011, Springer Science, New-York, NY 453–528.
12. Nucci MR. Uterine mesenchymal tumors. In: Crum CP, Lee KR, editors. Diagnostic gynecology and obstetric pathology. 2nd ed. Philadelphia, PA: Saunders Elsevier; 2011. p. 582–639.
13. Garcia L, Isaacson K. Adenomyosis: review of the literature. J Minim Invasive Gynecol. 2011;18(4):428–37.
14. Taran FA, Stewart EA, Brucker S. Adenomyosis: epidemiology, risk factors, clinical phenotype and surgical and interventional alternatives to hysterectomy. Geburtshilfe Frauenheilkd. 2013;73(9):924–31.
15. Vercellini P, et al. Adenomyosis: epidemiological factors. Best Pract Res Clin Obstet Gynaecol. 2006;20(4):465–77.
16. Ryan GL, Stolpen A, Van Voorhis BJ. An unusual cause of adolescent dysmenorrhea. Obstet Gynecol. 2006;108(4):1017–22.
17. Parker JD, et al. Persistence of dysmenorrhea and nonmenstrual pain after optimal endometriosis surgery may indicate adenomyosis. Fertil Steril. 2006;86(3):711–5.
18. Templeman C, et al. Adenomyosis and endometriosis in the California teachers study. Fertil Steril. 2008;90(2):415–24.
19. Weiss G, et al. Adenomyosis a variant, not a disease? Evidence from hysterectomized menopausal women in the study of Women's health across the nation (SWAN). Fertil Steril. 2009;91(1):201–6.
20. Vercellini P, et al. Adenomyosis at hysterectomy: a study on frequency distribution and patient characteristics. Hum Reprod. 1995;10(5):1160–2.
21. Parazzini F, et al. Risk factors for adenomyosis. Hum Reprod. 1997;12(6):1275–9.
22. Panganamamula UR, et al. Is prior uterine surgery a risk factor for adenomyosis? Obstet Gynecol. 2004;104(5 Pt 1):1034–8.
23. Curtis KM, et al. Disruption of the endometrial-myometrial border during pregnancy as a risk factor for adenomyosis. Am J Obstet Gynecol. 2002;187(3):543–4.
24. Guo SW, The Pathogenesis of Adenomyosis vis-a-vis endometriosis. J Clin Med. 2020;9(2):485.
25. Bergholt T, et al. Prevalence and risk factors of adenomyosis at hysterectomy. Hum Reprod. 2001;16(11):2418–21.
26. Taran FA, et al. Characteristics indicating adenomyosis coexisting with leiomyomas: a case-control study. Hum Reprod. 2010;25(5):1177–82.
27. Parazzini F, et al. Risk factors for adenomyosis. Hum Reprod (Oxford, England). 1997;12(6):1279–5.
28. Lacheta J. Uterine adenomyosis: pathogenesis, diagnostics, symptomatology and treatment. Ceska Gynekol. 2019;84(3):240–6.
29. Wainer R. Smoking and ovarian fertility. Gynecol Obstet Fertil. 2001;29(12):881–7.
30. Van Voorhis BJ, et al. The effects of smoking on ovarian function and fertility during assisted reproduction cycles. Obstet Gynecol. 1996;88(5):785–91.
31. Yeniel O, et al. Adenomyosis: prevalence, risk factors, symptoms and clinical findings. Clin Exp Obstet Gynecol. 2007;34(3):163–7.
32. Li X, Liu X, Guo SW. Clinical profiles of 710 premenopausal women with adenomyosis who underwent hysterectomy. J Obstet Gynaecol Res. 2014;40(2):485–94.
33. Kissler S, et al. Duration of dysmenorrhoea and extent of adenomyosis visualised by magnetic resonance imaging. Eur J Obstet Gynecol Reprod Biol. 2008;137(2):204–9.

34. Harel Z. Dysmenorrhea in adolescents and young adults: from pathophysiology to pharmacological treatments and management strategies. Expert Opin Pharmacother. 2008;9(15):2661–72.
35. Quinn M. Uterine innervation in adenomyosis. J Obstet Gynaecol. 2007;27(3):287–91.
36. Leyendecker G, et al. Adenomyosis and endometriosis. Re-visiting their association and further insights into the mechanisms of auto-traumatisation. An MRI study. Arch Gynecol Obstet. 2015;291(4):917–32.
37. Naftalin J, et al. Is adenomyosis associated with menorrhagia? Hum Reprod. 2014;29(3):473–9.
38. Gordts S, Grimbizis G, Campo R. Symptoms and classification of uterine adenomyosis, including the place of hysteroscopy in diagnosis. Fertil Steril. 2018;109(3):380–388.e1.
39. McCausland AM. Hysteroscopic myometrial biopsy: its use in diagnosing adenomyosis and its clinical application. Am J Obstet Gynecol. 1992;166(6 Pt 1):1619–26. discussion 1626-8
40. Munro MG, et al. FIGO classification system (PALM-COEIN) for causes of abnormal uterine bleeding in nongravid women of reproductive age. Int J Gynaecol Obstet. 2011;113(1):3–13.
41. Pervez SN, Javed K. Adenomyosis among samples from hysterectomy due to abnormal uterine bleeding. J Ayub Med Coll Abbottabad. 2013;25(1–2):68–70.
42. Mobarakeh MD, Maghsudi A, Rashidi I. Adenomyosis among samples from hysterectomy due to abnormal uterine bleeding in Ahwaz, southern Iran. Adv Biomed Res. 2012;1:49.
43. Younes G, Tulandi T. Effects of adenomyosis on in vitro fertilization treatment outcomes: a meta-analysis. Fertil Steril. 2017;108(3):483–490.e3.
44. Salim R, et al. Adenomyosis reduces pregnancy rates in infertile women undergoing IVF. Reprod Biomed Online. 2012;25(3):273–7.
45. Vercellini P, et al. Uterine adenomyosis and in vitro fertilization outcome: a systematic review and meta-analysis. Hum Reprod. 2014;29(5):964–77.
46. Peric H, Fraser IS. The symptomatology of adenomyosis. Best Pract Res Clin Obstet Gynaecol. 2006;20(4):547–55.
47. Champaneria R, et al. Ultrasound scan and magnetic resonance imaging for the diagnosis of adenomyosis: systematic review comparing test accuracy. Acta Obstet Gynecol Scand. 2010;89(11):1374–84.
48. Sofic A, et al. The significance of MRI evaluation of the uterine Junctional zone in the early diagnosis of Adenomyosis. Acta Inform Med. 2016;24(2):103–6.
49. Kishi Y, et al. Four subtypes of adenomyosis assessed by magnetic resonance imaging and their specification. Am J Obstet Gynecol. 2012;207(2):114.e1–7.
50. Grimbizis GF, Mikos T, Tarlatzis B. Uterus-sparing operative treatment for adenomyosis. Fertil Steril. 2014;101(2):472–87. e8
51. Bazot M, Darai E. Role of transvaginal sonography and magnetic resonance imaging in the diagnosis of uterine adenomyosis. Fertil Steril. 2018;109(3):389–97.
52. Babacan A, et al. CA 125 and other tumor markers in uterine leiomyomas and their association with lesion characteristics. Int J Clin Exp Med. 2014;7(4):1078–83.
53. Kil K, et al. Usefulness of CA125 in the differential diagnosis of uterine adenomyosis and myoma. Eur J Obstet Gynecol Reprod Biol. 2015;185:131–5.
54. El-Toukhy T, et al. Hysteroscopy in recurrent in-vitro fertilisation failure (TROPHY): a multicentre, randomised controlled trial. Lancet. 2016;387(10038):2614–21.

Adenomyosis and Pain

Xiaoyan Li, Shan Deng, and Jinhua Leng

Adenomyosis affects about 20% of women of reproductive age and is responsible for menorrhagia, dysmenorrhea, menstrual pelvic pain, dyspareunia, and infertility [1]. The causes of adenomyosis-related pain are unclear. When combined with endometriosis, especially deep infiltrating endometriosis (DIE), dysmenorrhea is more severe in patients with adenomyosis, and the chance of progressive dysmenorrhea will increase. Other pain mechanisms related to adenomyosis include abnormal uterine contractility and abnormal expression of the oxytocin receptor (OTR), abnormal expression of prostaglandin (PG) and cyclooxygenase 2 (COX-2), abnormal growth and distribution of local nerve fibers, neuropeptides, macrophages, abnormal secretion of cells and inflammatory factors, and so on. There may still be some unknown mechanisms that need further study and research.

5.1 Clinical Characteristics

The most common clinical manifestation of adenomyosis is pain, which mainly exists in the form of dysmenorrhea. Ultrasound examination for young women between 18 and 30 years of age suffering from dysmenorrhea showed a 34% incidence of adenomyosis and is associated with dysmenorrhea [2]. Adenomyosis-induced pain often occurs during the menstrual period, moreover at the uterine area, more than other endometriosis sites; its pain is severe. It is the first main reason for patients to seek medical treatment [3].

The International Association for the Study of Pain defines pain as "an unpleasant sensory and emotional experience associated with actual or potential tissue damage or described in terms of such damage." The complaint of dysmenorrhea in

X. Li · S. Deng · J. Leng (✉)
Department of Obstetrics and Gynecology, Peking Union Medical College Hospital, Beijing, China

© The Author(s), under exclusive license to Springer Nature Singapore Pte Ltd. 2021
M. Xue et al. (eds.), *Adenomyosis*, https://doi.org/10.1007/978-981-33-4095-4_5

women with adenomyosis is more often than any other gynecological diseases [4, 5]. It is the leading cause of gynecological morbidity in young Asian women, regardless of age, race, and economic status [6]. They are so-called secondary dysmenorrhea, which is mainly due to endometriosis and adenomyosis. In young women, this complaint is often unresponsive or partially responsive to non-steroidal anti-inflammatory drugs or to oral contraceptives. Some women with adenomyosis have very severe pain, severe enough to render them requiring absence from school or work. They suffered severely painful cramps occurring over several days every month, persisting for decades. Moreover, previous reports showed that adenomyosis negatively impacts daily activities and the quality of life of the affected women, with a subsequent increase in the risk of anxiety, depression, and other psychological disorders [7–9]. Then, it ends up reducing individual women to work and socialize in society, resulting annually in an important loss of productivity [6]. Therefore, the World Health Organization concluded that dysmenorrhea is probably the most important cause of chronic pelvic pain [10].

Clinical presentation of adenomyosis can vary, with mild adenomyosis that can be highly symptomatic, whereas others with very enlarged uteri due to adenomyosis may present only with mild symptoms. One-third of women with adenomyosis are asymptomatic [11]. Although the association of adenomyosis with dysmenorrhea is still debatable, the reported incidence of dysmenorrhea in adenomyosis was reported to be between 50 and 93.4% [12, 13]. A linear correlation had also been described between the extent of the adenomyosis and the severity of dysmenorrhea [14].

5.2 Pain Mechanisms of Adenomyosis

5.2.1 Related to Endometriosis

Adenomyosis often associates with concomitant diseases that have similar symptomatology, and it thus masks the causal relationship between the disease and its symptoms. For patients with adenomyosis, the most frequent coexisting morbidities are endometriosis and fibroids [15].

About 24.6–80.6% of adenomyosis patients are associated with endometriosis [16, 17], and both conditions share the same pathogenesis and symptoms, such as dysmenorrhea, heavy menstrual bleeding, infertility, dyspareunia, and chronic pelvic pain [18–20]. It is also well-defined that there is an overlap in the pathogenesis of DIE and adenomyosis [21, 22]. These patients with both conditions had a higher rate of a moderate-to-severe degree of dysmenorrhea (60.0% vs. 39.3%, $P = 0.001$) and a higher percentage of progressively worsening dysmenorrhea (47.8% vs. 32.0%, $P = 0.007$). [23]. If associated with DIE, the severity of dysmenorrhea is more apparently related to the extent of infiltrating endometriosis. In patients with DIE, the prevalence of adenomyosis is 48.7–66.3% [24, 25]. There is a statistically significant correlation between pelvic pain and the presence of adenomyosis, in agreement with the previously reported results [26]. When patients had both DIE and adenomyosis, 95.5% described the pain intensity of dysmenorrhea as severe while that of dyspareunia and dysuria moderate to severe [27–29].

Focal adenomyosis of the outer myometrium was more frequently found in endometriosis-affected women, especially those with deep endometriosis [25], and it supports the hypothesis of different pathogenesis between the inner and outer myometrium forms of adenomyosis [30].

In some studies, women with adenomyosis were found to have a higher incidence of dysmenorrhea than those with fibroids, only with an odds ratio of 3.4 (95% CI 1.8–6.4) [13, 15]. A retrospective study showed that women with adenomyosis had 4.5 folds more of having endometriosis compared with women with fibroids [31]. Therefore patients with symptomatic uterine fibroids should be wary of having associated adenomyosis at the same time.

5.2.2 Related to Anatomical Factors

The uterine myometrium has two layers of structures, (1) the outer myometrium and (2) the inner myometrium. The latter is also known as the sub-endometrial layer or endometrial–myometrial junctional zone (JZ). The JZ is just next to the endometrium and also undergoes cycle-dependent changes. It is from the Mullerian origin, while the outer myometrium is from the mesenchymal origin [32]. The dysperistaltic uterine contraction of the JZ in patients with endometriosis and adenomyosis can result in a more retrograde menstruation and a disturbed tubal sperm transport [33].

First, in terms of the depth of infiltration of adenomyosis, some authors suggested that the severity of symptoms and the clinical features correlated with the extent and depth of the infiltration [19, 34]. Bird et al. 1972 [35] reported that dysmenorrhea was present in 4.3% of women whose uterus had histologically defined grade I penetration and in 42.4% and 83.3% of women with grade II and grade III penetration, respectively. Second, the number of adenomyosis lesions was closely related to the patient's symptoms. Levgur et al. 2000 [36] reported a positive correlation between the number of ultrasound features of adenomyosis and the severity of dysmenorrhea. The relationship between the number of histopathology features and clinical manifestations had been clarified in previous studies on specimens obtained from hysterectomies. These studies confirmed the direct correlation of adenomyotic foci number with severe dysmenorrhea [36–38]. Based on these findings, the hypothesis of a causal relationship was established between the number and depth of infiltration of the adenomyotic and specific symptoms.

5.3 Related to Molecular Mechanisms

5.3.1 Prostaglandins and Cyclooxygenase 2

The molecular mechanisms of dysmenorrhea and pelvic pain in women with adenomyosis are not well-understood, but PG may play an important role [39].

Although PG could excite nociceptors and cause pain, it is believed that PG indirectly cause cramping pain by stimulating uterine contractility [40], thus causing abnormal contraction of the uterus and increased contraction. Some previous studies had reported that PGF2α administration increased uterine contractility and elicited visceral pain. Drugs that inhibit PG syntheses, such as ibuprofen and naproxen, reduce uterine contractility in dysmenorrheic women [41]. It has been suggested that PG produced cramping pain via temporary elevations in uterine pressure. However, not all women with dysmenorrhea have alterations in uterine pressure; other mechanisms might have contributed to the menstrual pain, for example, reduced uterine blood flow, myometrial ischemia, and hypoxia [42].

Preclinical research studies suggested that PG-dependent mechanisms cause dysmenorrhea in majority of women [43]. The breakdown of endometrial tissues frees phospholipids from the cellular membrane. Uterine phospholipases convert the available phospholipids into arachidonic acid, which is then synthesized into PG via cyclooxygenase (COX)-1 and -2. COX-2 is a key enzyme in the process of synthesis of various endogenous PG. COX-2 has certain associations with inflammation, cell mitosis, and specific signaling transduction pathways. The level of PG in the peritoneal fluid of patients with endometriosis or adenomyosis is significantly increased compared with those without these diseases. It is positively associated with the severity of dysmenorrhea. Therefore non-steroidal anti-inflammatory drugs can effectively relieve pain [44, 45]. Notably, COX-2 expression is highest during menses, and the end products prostaglandin E2 (PGE2) and PGF2α are elevated in the menstrual effluent in dysmenorrheic women with adenomyosis when compared with healthy controls [46, 47].

5.3.2 Abnormality of Uterine Contraction and Oxytocin/ Vasopressin Receptors

It is well-known that oxytocin can cause painful contraction of the uterine smooth muscle. The expression of OTR in the ectopic endometrial glands and interstitial tissues was significantly increased and was positively correlated with the degree of dysmenorrhea [55]. Uterine hyperperistalsis and the increased expression levels of OTR in patients with adenomyosis may contribute to the severity of dysmenorrhea. Mechsner et al. 2010 [48] in their immunohistochemical study of both OTR and vasopressin receptor (VP1αR) expression in the endometrium, myometrium, and adenomyotic lesions demonstrated that overexpression of OTR was in the adenomyosis-surrounding myometrium, while overexpression of VP1αR was in the myometrial cells and blood vessels. These specific receptor expressions in the myometrial tissues suggested that the induced dysperistalsis played an essential role in the development of dysmenorrhea in patients with adenomyosis.

5.3.3   Other Inflammatory Factors

The local immune response in patients with adenomyosis can lead to the production of cytokines and the release of inflammatory factors from the ectopic endometrial lesions that influence the severity of pain. Hyperestrogenism is common in patients with adenomyosis and can stimulate the production of cytokines [49]. Local inflammation is involved in the pathogenesis of dysmenorrhea in adenomyosis because of the high expression of interleukin 1β, corticotropin-releasing hormone (CRH) and urocortin (UCN), and nerve growth factors (NGFs) in adenomyotic lesions [50]. Local production of interleukin-1 (IL-1) is due to tissue traumatization and healing, and it also induces the COX-2 enzyme, causing PGE2 production. The high levels of CRH and UCN in adenomyosis are also involved in increased PG synthesis [50].

5.3.4   Nerve Fibers

It has been reported that patients with endometriosis and dysmenorrhea have a greater tendency to stimulate the release of NGFs, and patients with endometriosis can release these growth factors to lead nerve fiber growth into ectopic lesions [51]. The myometrium is innervated by a subserosal nerve plexus and a plexus at the endometrial–myometrial junction [52]. Sensory unmyelinated C nerve fibers innervate the endometrium, and inflammatory mediators released from the endometrium may activate or sensitize these nerve fibers, resulting in neurogenic inflammation. As a result, PGE2, prostacyclin, and norepinephrine will be released from adrenergic fiber endings, which then affect sensory C [53] pain fibers. Post-hysterectomy specimens showed the focal proliferation of small-diameter nerve fibers at the margins of adenomyosis in some uteri [54]. Zhang et al. 2010 [55] studied nerve fiber density in women with painful adenomyosis by using protein gene product (PGP) 9.5 immunostaining; they found that nerve fiber density was significantly increased in the basal layer of the endometrium and myometrium. They believed that these nerve fibers might play a role in pain generation in adenomyosis. Lertvikool et al. 2014 [56] also studied the nerve fiber density in adenomyosis tissue with both PGP 9.5 and neurofilament (NF) immunostainings; they found that nerve fiber density was significantly increased in women with adenomyosis experiencing moderate and severe pain as compared with those experiencing mild pain. Therefore it showed a good correlation between the severity of dysmenorrhea and the concentration of nerve fibers in adenomyosis specimens. Choi et al. 2015 [57] found a higher NF expression in the endometrium and the lesions of adenomyosis. They assumed that NF-positive cells might play a role in the pathogenesis of adenomyosis.

5.3.5   Neurogenic Factors

Nerve growth factor is reported to be involved in pain, neural plasticity, immune cell aggregation, and release of inflammatory factors. The increase of NGF-β and its receptor levels when the adenomyosis worsens suggests a role of NGF-β in adenomyosis pathogenesis [58].

CD56, a neural cell adhesion molecule (NCAM) is expressed in neural tissues, neuroendocrine tissues, and tumors; it is involved with the growth and aggregation of nerve fibers and neuroendocrine tumor metastases [59]. In endometriosis, increased CD56 was found in the interstitial tissue of endometriotic foci, suggesting that endometriosis-related pain may be due to increased nerve fiber density, which leads to hyperalgesia in the interstitium [60]. Wang et al. 2015 [61] found that CD56 was mainly expressed in the endometrial glandular epithelium. Its CD56 immunostaining intensity in the ectopic endometrium of patients with adenomyosis was found positively correlated with the severity of dysmenorrhea. Because CD56 increases the sensitivity and density of local nerve fibers, patients who have high CD56 expression in the adenomyotic tissue are more likely to suffer from dysmenorrhea than those who have low expression.

Additionally, estrogen and progesterone receptors have been detected in adenomyotic tissues, and estradiol is known to increase the expression of CD56, whereas progesterone treatment suppresses estradiol-induced gene expression of CD56 [62]. This evidence may partly explain the cyclic variation of CD56 expression in the eutopic endometrium of adenomyosis.

As in previous studies of adenomyosis, macrophages were detected not only in adenomyosis but also in large enough numbers in the myometrium, around the major blood vessels and in the stroma between bundles of the smooth muscle cells. These nerve fibers in the myometrium and the eutopic endometrium can be stimulated by inflammatory humoral factors, including histamine, serotonin, bradykinin, PG, leukotriene, etc., that cause increased pain. Macrophages themselves secrete many of the above substances. Therefore increasing macrophages and their secreted algogenic (pain-inducing) factors are possible causes of pain in women with adenomyosis and endometriosis [63]. There is also strong evidence that macrophages are important in the regeneration process of nerve fibers in the peripheral nervous system and involve the inflammation of nerve terminals in the myometrium. In adenomyosis, local inflammation is also accompanied by the release of various algogenic factors and changes of nociceptors and causes an increase in their excitability [64]. When the functions of macrophages are disrupted, the regeneration of sensory nerve fibers is reduced. Therefore, the viability and repair of the nerve fibers depend on many factors whose products are regulated by activated macrophages [65]. Adenomyosis is known as a chronic inflammatory disease, which is accompanied by an abnormal immune reactivity in the myometrium. An increase in the number of activated macrophages in the perivascular compartments and areas of the myometrium leads to a vicious cycle of increased neurogenic inflammation and hypersensitivity of nociceptors, activation of peripheral nerve fibers. It serves as the main pathogenetic mechanism of the formation of chronic pelvic pain in women with adenomyosis [66].

To summarize, there is no commonly accepted mechanism to account for adenomyosis-induced menstrual pain and chronic pelvic pain. There are still many uncertainties about the cause and mechanism of adenomyosis pain. For example, why the presence of an irregular endometrial–myometrial junction should be associated with painful periods and so on? As pain can seriously affect the quality of life of patients with adenomyosis, these findings do suggest some directions of future research to investigate the mechanisms of pain in adenomyosis. When the characteristics of adenomyosis pain are sufficiently understood, diagnosis and differential diagnosis may be made when there are early symptoms. Then early intervention can be achieved, and the medication and treatment of pain in adenomyosis may be more accurate.

References

1. Donnez J, Donnez O, Dolmans MM. Introduction: uterine adenomyosis, another enigmatic disease of our time. Fertil Steril. 2018;109(3):369–70.
2. Wise SS. Management of perioperative pain. Surgery: Springer; 2008. p. 381–93.
3. Bernardi M, Lazzeri L, Perelli F, Reis FM, Petraglia F. Dysmenorrhea and related disorders. F1000Research. 2017;6:1645.
4. Patel V, Tanksale V, Sahasrabhojanee M, Gupte S, Nevrekar P. The burden and determinants of dysmenorrhoea: a population-based survey of 2262 women in Goa, India. BJOG. 2006;113(4):453–63.
5. Desai S, Shuka A, Nambiar D, Ved R. Patterns of hysterectomy in India: a national and state-level analysis of the fourth National Family Health Survey (2015-2016). BJOG. 2019;126(Suppl 4):72–80.
6. Wong LP, Khoo EM. Dysmenorrhea in a multiethnic population of adolescent Asian girls. Int J Gynecol Obstet. 2010;108(2):139–42.
7. Culley L, Law C, Hudson N, Denny E, Mitchell H, Baumgarten M, et al. The social and psychological impact of endometriosis on women's lives: a critical narrative review. Hum Reprod Update. 2013;19(6):625–39.
8. Pluchino N, Wenger J-M, Petignat P, Tal R, Bolmont M, Taylor HS, et al. Sexual function in endometriosis patients and their partners: effect of the disease and consequences of treatment. Hum Reprod Update. 2016;22(6):762–74.
9. Bernardi M, Lazzeri L, Perelli F, Reis FM, Petraglia F. Dysmenorrhea and related disorders. F1000Res. 2017;6:1645.
10. Eryilmaz G, Ozdemir F, Pasinlioglu T. Dysmenorrhea prevalence among adolescents in eastern Turkey: its effects on school performance and relationships with family and friends. J Pediatr Adolesc Gynecol. 2010;23(5):267–72.
11. 中华医学会妇产科学分会子宫内膜异位症协作组. 子宫内膜异位症的诊治指南. 中华妇产科杂志. 2015(3).
12. Li X, Liu X, Guo S-W. Clinical profiles of 710 premenopausal women with adenomyosis who underwent hysterectomy. J Obstet Gynaecol Res. 2014;40(2):485–94.
13. Taran FA, Wallwiener M, Kabashi D, Rothmund R, Rall K, Kraemer B, et al. Clinical characteristics indicating adenomyosis at the time of hysterectomy: a retrospective study in 291 patients. Arch Gynecol Obstet. 2012;285(6):1571–6.
14. Kissler S, Zangos S, Kohl J, Wiegratz I, Rody A, Gätje R, et al. Duration of dysmenorrhoea and extent of adenomyosis visualised by magnetic resonance imaging. Eur J Obstet Gynecol Reprod Biol. 2008;137(2):204–9.
15. Nezhat C, Li A, Abed S, Balassiano E, Soliemannjad R, Nezhat A, et al. Strong association between endometriosis and symptomatic leiomyomas. JSLS: Journal of the Society of Laparoendoscopic Surgeons. 2016;20(3):e2016.00053.
16. Leyendecker G, Bilgicyildirim A, Inacker M, Stalf T, Huppert P, Mall G, et al. Adenomyosis and endometriosis. Re-visiting their association and further insights into the mechanisms of auto-traumatisation. An MRI study. Arch Gynecol Obstet. 2015;291(4):917–32.

17. Larsen SB, Lundorf E, Forman A, Dueholm M. Adenomyosis and junctional zone changes in patients with endometriosis. Eur J Obstet Gynecol Reprod Biol. 2011;157(2):206–11.
18. Alabiso G, Alio L, Arena S, Barbasetti di Prun A, Bergamini V, Berlanda N, et al. Adenomyosis: what the patient needs. J Minim Invasive Gynecol. 2016;23(4):476–88.
19. Vercellini P, Consonni D, Dridi D, Bracco B, Frattaruolo MP, Somigliana E. Uterine adenomyosis and in vitro fertilization outcome: a systematic review and meta-analysis. Hum Reprod. 2014;29(5):964–77.
20. Onchee Y, Schulze-Rath R, Grafton MJ, Hansen MK, Scholes D. Adenomyosis incidence, prevalence and treatment: United States population based study 2006–2015. Am J Obstet Gynecol. 2020;223(1):94.e1–94.e10.
21. Brosens I, Kunz G, Benagiano G. Is adenomyosis the neglected phenotype of an endomyometrial dysfunction syndrome? Gynecol Surg. 2012;9(2):131–7.
22. Pinzauti S, Lazzeri L, Tosti C, Centini G, Orlandini C, Luisi S, et al. Transvaginal sonographic features of diffuse adenomyosis in 18-30-year-old nulligravid women without endometriosis: association with symptoms. Ultrasound Obstet Gynecol: the official journal of the International Society of Ultrasound in Obstetrics and Gynecology. 2015;46(6):730–6.
23. Chen Q, Li YW, Wang S, Fan QB, Shi HH, Leng JH, et al. Clinical manifestations of Adenomyosis patients with or without pain symptoms. J Pain Res. 2019;12:3127–33.
24. Lazzeri L, Di Giovanni A, Exacoustos C, Tosti C, Pinzauti S, Malzoni M, et al. Preoperative and postoperative clinical and transvaginal ultrasound findings of adenomyosis in patients with deep infiltrating endometriosis. Reprod Sci (Thousand Oaks, Calif). 2014;21(8):1027–33.
25. Chapron C, Tosti C, Marcellin L, Bourdon M, Lafay-Pillet M-C, Millischer A-E, et al. Relationship between the magnetic resonance imaging appearance of adenomyosis and endometriosis phenotypes. Human Reprod (Oxford, England). 2017;32(7):1393–401.
26. Vercellini P, Viganò P, Somigliana E, Daguati R, Abbiati A, Fedele L. Adenomyosis: epidemiological factors. Best Pract Res Clin Obstet Gynaecol. 2006;20(4):465–77.
27. Bazot M, Fiori O, Darai E. Adenomyosis in endometriosis--prevalence and impact on fertility. Evidence from magnetic resonance imaging. Human Reprod (Oxford, England). 2006;21(4):1101–2.
28. Perello MF, Martinez-Zamora MA, Torres X, Munros J, Balasch Cortina J, Carmona F. Endometriotic pain is associated with Adenomyosis but not with the compartments affected by deep infiltrating endometriosis. Gynecol Obstet Investig. 2017;82(3):240–6.
29. Haas D, Oppelt P, Shebl O, Shamiyeh A, Schimetta W, Mayer R. Enzian classification: does it correlate with clinical symptoms and the rASRM score? Acta Obstet Gynecol Scand. 2013;92(5):562–6.
30. Kishi Y, Suginami H, Kuramori R, Yabuta M, Suginami R, Taniguchi F. Four subtypes of adenomyosis assessed by magnetic resonance imaging and their specification. Am J Obstet Gynecol. 2012;207(2):114.e1–7.
31. Taran FA, Weaver AL, Coddington CC, Stewart EA. Understanding adenomyosis: a case control study. Fertil Steril. 2010;94(4):1223–8.
32. Noe M, Kunz G, Herbertz M, Mall G, Leyendecker G. The cyclic pattern of the immunocytochemical expression of oestrogen and progesterone receptors in human myometrial and endometrial layers: characterization of the endometrial-subendometrial unit. Human Reprod (Oxford, England). 1999;14(1):190–7.
33. Kissler S, Siebzehnruebl E, Kohl J, Mueller A, Hamscho N, Gaetje R, et al. Uterine contractility and directed sperm transport assessed by hysterosalpingoscintigraphy (HSSG) and intrauterine pressure (IUP) measurement. Acta Obstet Gynecol Scand. 2004;83(4):369–74.
34. Bergeron C, Amant F, Ferenczy A. Pathology and physiopathology of adenomyosis. Best Pract Res Clin Obstet Gynaecol. 2006;20(4):511–21.
35. Bird CC, McElin TW, Manalo-Estrella P. The elusive adenomyosis of the uterus—revisited. Am J Obstet Gynecol. 1972;112(5):583–93.
36. Levgur M, Abadi MA, Tucker A. Adenomyosis: symptoms, histology, and pregnancy terminations. Obstet Gynecol. 2000;95(5):688–91.

37. Bird CC, McElin TW, Manalo-Estrella P. The elusive adenomyosis of the uterus--revisited. Am J Obstet Gynecol. 1972;112(5):583–93.
38. Nishida M. Relationship between the onset of dysmenorrhea and histologic findings in adenomyosis. Am J Obstet Gynecol. 1991;165(1):229–31.
39. Harel Z. Dysmenorrhea in adolescents and young adults: from pathophysiology to pharmacological treatments and management strategies. Expert Opin Pharmacother. 2008;9(15):2661–72.
40. Dawood MY. Primary dysmenorrhea: advances in pathogenesis and management. Obstet Gynecol. 2006;108(2):428–41.
41. Oladosu FA, Tu FF, Hellman KM. Nonsteroidal antiinflammatory drug resistance in dysmenorrhea: epidemiology, causes, and treatment. Am J Obstet Gynecol. 2018;218(4):390–400.
42. Oladosu FA, Tu FF, Hellman KM. Nonsteroidal antiinflammatory drug resistance in dysmenorrhea: epidemiology, causes, and treatment. Am J Obstet Gynecol. 2018;218(4):390–400.
43. Maia H, Maltez A, Studard E, Zausner B, Athayde C, Coutinho E. Effect of the menstrual cycle and oral contraceptives on cyclooxygenase-2 expression in the endometrium. Gynecol Endocrinol: the official journal of the International Society of Gynecological Endocrinology. 2005;21(1):57–61.
44. Lousse JC, Defrère S, Colette S, Van Langendonckt A, Donnez J. Expression of eicosanoid biosynthetic and catabolic enzymes in peritoneal endometriosis. Human Reprod (Oxford, England). 2010;25(3):734–41.
45. Li C, Chen R, Jiang C, Chen L, Cheng Z. Correlation of LOX5 and COX2 expression with inflammatory pathology and clinical features of adenomyosis. Mol Med Rep. 2019;19(1):727–33.
46. Chan WY. Prostaglandins and nonsteroidal antiinflammatory drugs in dysmenorrhea. Annu Rev Pharmacol Toxicol. 1983;23:131–49.
47. Lundström V, Gréen K. Endogenous levels of prostaglandin F2alpha and its main metabolites in plasma and endometrium of normal and dysmenorrheic women. Am J Obstet Gynecol. 1978;130(6):640–6.
48. Mechsner S, Grum B, Gericke C, Loddenkemper C, Dudenhausen JW, Ebert AD. Possible roles of oxytocin receptor and vasopressin 1α receptor in the pathomechanism of dysperistalsis and dysmenorrhea in patients with adenomyosis uteri. Fertil Steril. 2010;94(7):2541–6.
49. Leyendecker G, Wildt L, Mall G. The pathophysiology of endometriosis and adenomyosis: tissue injury and repair. Arch Gynecol Obstet. 2009;280(4):529–38.
50. Carrarelli P, Yen C-F, Funghi L, Arcuri F, Tosti C, Bifulco G, et al. Expression of inflammatory and neurogenic mediators in adenomyosis: a pathogenetic role. Reprod Sci. 2017;24(3):369–75.
51. Mechsner S, Schwarz J, Thode J, Loddenkemper C, Salomon DS, Ebert AD. Growth-associated protein 43-positive sensory nerve fibers accompanied by immature vessels are located in or near peritoneal endometriotic lesions. Fertil Steril. 2007;88(3):581–7.
52. Krantz KE. Innervation of the human uterus. Ann N Y Acad Sci. 1959;75:770–84.
53. Apfel SC. Neurotrophic factors and pain. Clin J Pain. 2000;16(2 Suppl):S7–11.
54. Quinn M Uterine innervation in adenomyosis. (0144–3615 (Print)).
55. Zhang X, Lu B, Huang X, Xu H, Zhou C, Lin J. Innervation of endometrium and myometrium in women with painful adenomyosis and uterine fibroids. Fertil Steril. 2010;94(2):730–7.
56. Lertvikool S, Sukprasert M, Pansrikaew P, Rattanasiri S, Weerakiet S. Comparative study of nerve fiber density between adenomyosis patients with moderate to severe pain and mild pain. J Med Assoc Thai Chotmaihet Thangphaet. 2014;97(8):791–7.
57. Choi YJ, Chang J-A, Kim YA, Chang SH, Chun KC, Koh JW. Innervation in women with uterine myoma and adenomyosis. Obstet Gynecol Sci. 2015;58(2):150–6.
58. Li Y, Zhang S-f, Zou S-e, Bao L. Accumulation of nerve growth factor and its receptors in the uterus and dorsal root ganglia in a mouse model of adenomyosis. Reprod Biol Endocrinol. 2011;9:30. https://doi.org/10.1186/1477-7827-9-30. (1477–7827 (Electronic))
59. Kleene R, Mzoughi M, Joshi G, Kalus I, Bormann U, Schulze C, et al. NCAM-induced neurite outgrowth depends on binding of calmodulin to NCAM and on nuclear import of NCAM and fak fragments. J Neurosci. 2010;30(32):10784–98.

60. Odagiri K, Konno R, Fujiwara H, Netsu S, Yang C, Suzuki M. Smooth muscle metapla-
    sia and innervation in interstitium of endometriotic lesions related to pain. Fertil Steril.
    2009;92(5):1525–31.
61. Wang F, Shi X, Qin X, Wen Z, Zhao X, Li C. Expression of CD56 in patients with adeno-
    myosis and its correlation with dysmenorrhea. European J Obstet Gynecol Reprod Biology.
    2015;194:101–5.
62. Bethea CL, Reddy AP. Effect of ovarian steroids on gene expression related to synapse assem-
    bly in serotonin neurons of macaques. J Neurosci Res. 2012;90(7):1324–34. (1097–4547
    (Electronic))
63. Tran LVP, Tokushige N, Berbic M, Markham R, Fraser IS. Macrophages and nerve fibres in
    peritoneal endometriosis. Hum Reprod. 2009;24(4):835–41.
64. Moalem G, Tracey DJ. Immune and inflammatory mechanisms in neuropathic pain. Brain
    Res Rev. 2006;51(2):240–64. https://doi.org/10.1016/j.brainresrev.2005.11.004. (0165–0173
    (Print))
65. Tran LV, Tokushige N, Berbic M, Markham R, Fraser IS. Macrophages and nerve fibres in
    peritoneal endometriosis. Hum Reprod. 2009;24(4):835–41. https://doi.org/10.1093/humrep/
    den483. (1460–2350 (Electronic))
66. Orazov MR, Radzinsky VE, Nosenko EN, Khamoshina MB, Dukhin AO, Lebedeva
    MG. Immune-inflammatory predictors of the pelvic pain syndrome associated with adeno-
    myosis. Gynecol Endocrinol. 2017;33(Supp 1):44–6.

Adenomyosis and Abnormal Uterine Bleeding

6

Shan Deng and Jinhua Leng

The complex pathogenesis and different manifestations of adenomyosis make it a difficult cause of abnormal uterine bleeding to be diagnosed and treated. Adenomyosis can be divided generally into three types: intrinsic, extrinsic, and intermediate. Different types have different clinical presentations. In terms of intrinsic type, the cause of abnormal uterine bleeding is more obvious, and dysmenorrhea may not occur at the same time. It is because the abnormal uterine bleeding may be closely related to abnormal angiogenesis or other factors. The uterine bleeding is characterized by heavy menstrual flow and irregular bleeding, which is often encountered even during drug treatment, such as placing levonorgestrel-releasing intrauterine system (LNG-IUS) or gonadotropin-releasing hormone antagonist (GnRHa) injection or taking dienogest. Magnetic resonance imaging (MRI) can guide the detailed classification of adenomyosis with refractory bleeding and the treatment options.

Adenomyosis is a visually objective structural disease in the FIGO PALM-COEIN classification of causes of abnormal uterine bleeding [1]. Its main symptom is heavy menstrual bleeding (about 60%) and pain (about 25%); about 1/3 of women with adenomyosis have no apparent symptoms.

With the in-depth exploration of the pathogenesis of adenomyosis and the progression of imaging, especially nuclear magnetic resonance, the ability to recognize different degrees/locations of lesions helps to refine the disease typing. It is speculated that the intrinsic and extrinsic types may originate from different germ layers of the uterine embryo development. In the past, adenomyosis and endometriosis were considered to be two independent diseases. However, in fact, there are many similarities in the clinical appearance and pathogenesis of two diseases, which may be largely caused by "eutopic endometrial determinism" of homogenous diseases [2].

S. Deng · J. Leng (✉)
Department of Obstetrics and Gynecology, Peking Union Medical College Hospital, Beijing, China

© The Author(s), under exclusive license to Springer Nature Singapore Pte Ltd. 2021
M. Xue et al. (eds.), *Adenomyosis*, https://doi.org/10.1007/978-981-33-4095-4_6

6.1   Clinical Manifestation

About a third of the patients with adenomyosis have no apparent symptoms. However, adenomyosis can cause heavy menstrual bleeding, irregular uterine bleeding, and abnormal uterine bleeding that do not respond well to conventional medications. In addition to pathological diagnosis, a specific transvaginal ultrasound and magnetic resonance imaging (MRI) can help to diagnose and type the adenomyosis lesions [3, 4]. Drugs can effectively control symptoms associated with adenomyosis. Medical treatment includes oral contraceptives, high-dose progestins, selective estrogen receptor modulators (SERMs), selective progesterone receptor modulators (SPRMs), LNG-IUS, an aromatase inhibitor, danazol, short-term GnRHa. As long as the purpose of amenorrhea can be achieved, there is no significant difference in the analgesic effect of various drugs; only the side effects and costs are different [5].

The consensus among doctors is that LNG-IUS is most useful for treating adenomyosis for heavy bleeding [6]. LNG-IUS can significantly reduce adenomyosis-related heavy menstrual bleeding and pain, and its effect is better than combined oral contraceptives (COCs) [7]. After the insertion of the LNG-IUS, a patient with adenomyosis will have a decrease of menstrual flow, reached a plateau in about 6 months; dysmenorrhea eased to plateau phase in 1 year, and these symptoms continued to soothe in the following 6 years [8]. In patients with enlarged uterine cavity, abnormal uterine contractility, and excessive menstruation, the probability of intrauterine device (IUD) expulsion is slightly higher than that of normal women. The cumulative expulsion rate in 12 months is 11% [9]. GnRH-a should be applied before placement, and it can significantly reduce the rate of IUD expulsion. For patients with uterine deformation caused by focal adenomyomas, hysteroscopy can be performed before placing LNG-IUS, which can effectively improve the continuation rate. LNG-IUS can be placed under ultrasound surveillance if necessary. Compared with non-adenomyosis/-endometriosis patients, the side effects of irregular vaginal bleeding are more common after placing LNG-IUS in patients with adenomyosis. However, in general, the adverse reactions of this bleeding pattern have gradually improved over time. Adequate communication and reassurance are best to improve the compliance and satisfaction of the patients [10]. In the case of satisfactory control of adenomyosis-related symptoms, patients can be reassured to be observed if there is no more excessive bleeding; time is the best treatment. Other drug interventions, like COCs, antifibrinolytic agents, and/or anti-inflammatory agents, can be attempted, but efficacy is uncertain.

On the other hand, if there is no satisfactory control of symptoms or no obvious improvement in side effect management, the causes should be checked accordingly. Alternative treatment should be considered if necessary. Nevertheless, hysterectomy is still the most reliable treatment for patients with adenomyosis who failed medical treatment.

6.2 Recent Progress

Without dysmenorrhea, adenomyosis-related abnormal uterine bleeding is often overlooked or underestimated. In the absence of other uterine pathology, adenomyosis can cause abnormal uterine bleeding in 27% to 65% of patients. Severe anemia due to menorrhagia is highly suggestive of the probability of adenomyosis, especially in nulliparous women. Adenomyosis varies widely in the extent and its location within the uterus. MRI provides better diagnostic capability compared with the transvaginal ultrasound scan by its increased ability to differentiate types of soft tissue [11]. Our experience confirmed that MRI could provide more specific details about important parameters of the adenomyosis, like the "affected area" (inner or outer myometrium), "localization" (anterior or posterior or fundus), "pattern" (diffuse or focal), "type" (muscular or cystic), and "volume or size", as objective images from different angles, especially for the symmetrical internal subtype. It is helpful for the surgeon to make clinical decisions.

In recent years, Kishi et al. 2012 [12] proposed the four subtypes of adenomyosis based on MRI features, i.e., Type 1. intrinsic, Type 2. extrinsic, Type 3. intramural adenomyosis, as well as a subtype that will not satisfy with the above. The classification system was refined and amplified by Bazot et al., 2018 [13], into internal, external adenomyosis, and adenomyomas. Intrinsic adenomyosis develops between the thickened junctional zone and healthy myometrium. While extrinsic adenomyosis is located in the outer layer of the uterus, the junctional zone is kept intact without aberrancy, and the healthy muscular myometrium is preserved in between the adenomyosis and the junctional zone. Among them, intrinsic adenomyosis comprised focal or multifocal, superficial asymmetric or symmetric, and diffuse asymmetric or symmetric subtypes. The clinical impression is that the intrinsic subtype is more likely to present with severe bleeding, and the extrinsic subtype presented severe dysmenorrhea. Then it has the potential to plan therapeutic strategy and to reflect the different natures of the pathogenesis of adenomyosis.

Adenomyosis in many patients is underdiagnosed mostly, because patients do not complain of dysmenorrhea, while ultrasound scans just suggest the thickening of the endometrium. Then MRI examination opens a new and more in-depth insight for us. For mild intrinsic adenomyosis, ultrasound is less sensitive than MRI [13]. Although a new ultrasound scoring system for uterine adenomyosis has been published recently [14], for adenomyosis, where the uterine volume is not enlarged and only the superficial myometrial layer is involved, ultrasound tends to miss the lesion. MRI helps in clarifying the classification. This MRI information is very helpful in analyzing any drug resistance to treatment and formulates the next treatment plan. Because of the above, though a transvaginal ultrasound scan is the first-line imaging technique currently used for the diagnosis of adenomyosis and it continues to improve itself, it is not the only investigation, where the MRI may be needed to help out in the management of adenomyosis.

Besides, a recent single-center cross-sectional survey in China showed that using FIGO PALM-COEIN classification for abnormal uterine bleeding for a statistical study, adenomyosis only accounted for 4.94% of patients in the same period [15]. It is estimated that a lot of abnormal uterine bleeding-adenomyosis (AUB-A) patients are scattered in other subgroups in the above federation international of gynecology and obstetrics (FIGO) AUB classification. However, one must consider that adenomyosis is often diagnosed based on pathological findings; the incidence rate in the population may be higher than this ratio. Likely, many adenomyosis patients are not being diagnosed, unless MRI is used more often to diagnose adenomyosis.

6.3 Treatment Options for AUB Due to Adenomyosis

6.3.1 Removal of the Endometrium

Endometrial ablation can be used for the treatment of patients with adenomyosis presented with heavy periods. However, adenomyosis itself is one of the high-risk factors for poor treatment results, with a failure rate of about 20% [16].

For symptomatic adenomyosis, which is resistant to drug therapy to dysmenorrhea and abnormal uterine bleeding, second-generation endometrial ablation could be a choice. Based on a longitudinal study by Philip et al. 2018 [17] with a 36-month follow-up, NovaSure® was effective in the treatment of heavy periods associated with adenomyosis for both the short and long term. However, the control of heavy bleeding decreased over time. Postoperatively, there was a significant reduction in abnormal bleeding in 40 patients (93%) in 6 months and persistent improvement in 29 patients (67.4%) in 3 years. A total of 11 patients (25.5%) experienced a recurrence of abnormal bleeding between 6 months and 3 years. However, 18 patients (41.9%) experienced amenorrhea 6 months after the procedure and 16 patients (37.2%) in 3 years. It may appear to be a good alternative to hysterectomy, especially in patients close to menopause. In this study with NovaSure, eight patients (19%) had a hysterectomy after NovaSure treatment. About 92% of patients were satisfied with the procedure, and no major postoperative complication was reported.

6.3.2 Uterine Artery Embolization (UAE)

After UAE treatment for more than 1 year, the symptom remission rate is 50% ~ 90% [18]. The treatment with uterine artery embolization will be elaborated in Chap. 12 in this book.

6.3.3 MRg/USg High-Intensity Focused Ultrasound (HIFU) Ablation

One year after MRgHIFU/USgHIFU treatment, the reduction in the bleeding was 25–66% [19]. The treatment with HIFU ablation will be elaborated in Chap. 13 to 16 in this book.

6.3.4 New Medical Treatment

Dienogest (Visanne) is a new type of progestin, approved for the treatment of endometriosis. Because endometriosis and adenomyosis have many similarities in pathogenesis and clinical characteristics, and often coexistent, dienogest is also used to relieve adenomyosis-related pain symptoms [20]. However, irregular bleeding is the most common adverse reaction during the use of dienogest. Although the rate of discontinuation is low (6%), the incidence of abnormal uterine bleeding is as high as 97% [21–23]. The risk factors for severe irregular bleeding are low-baseline Hb levels, high dysmenorrhea scores, high CA-125 levels, age < 38 years, uterine sagittal square area $\geq$ 48 cm^2, and lesions located in the lining of the uterus involving the junctional zone. It can be seen that the indication of dienogest for adenomyosis is to control pain but not suitable for abnormal uterine bleeding. It may even worsen bleeding symptoms. Retrospective cohort studies have shown that the use of compatible GnRHa can reduce the side effects of irregular bleeding, and sequential treatment with GnRHa + dienogest is beneficial to prevent recurrence of menstrual periods and dysmenorrhea [24]. Also, a small clinical trial had been conducted with the use of dienogest combined with microwave endometrial ablation and showed that this treatment was useful for treating uterine adenomyosis with menorrhagia and dysmenorrhea [25].

To summarize,

1. Dysmenorrhea is not an indispensable "signature symptom" of adenomyosis. No pain is not equal to no adenomyosis. Heavy menstrual bleeding that is significant enough to cause anemia is highly suggestive of adenomyosis, especially in nulliparous women.
2. When routine medications are ineffective in the treatment of abnormal uterine bleeding caused by ovulatory dysfunction and endometrial malignancy is excluded, adenomyosis is much probably the underlying contributor even for the patients who do not complain of dysmenorrhea.
3. Adenomyosis is a predictor of treatment failure of heavy bleeding in terms of LNG-IUS, Endometrial ablation, and even GnRHa.
4. According to MRI, the intrinsic subtype of adenomyosis may present more severe uterine bleeding.
5. New medical and surgical treatments, the latter with UAE or HIFU ablation, can offer an alternative treatment to hysterectomy.

References

1. Deneris A. PALM-COEIN nomenclature for abnormal uterine bleeding. J Midwifery Womens Health. 2016;61(3):376–9.
2. Cheng AS, Deng S. New advances in uterine adenomyosis from pathogenesis to drug selection. Chinese J Obstet Gynecol. 2019;54(6):421–24.

3. Cunningham RK, et al. Adenomyosis: a sonographic diagnosis. Radiographics. 2018;38(5):1576–89.
4. Reinhold C, et al. Diffuse adenomyosis: comparison of endovaginal US and MR imaging with histopathologic correlation. Radiology. 1996;199(1):151–8.
5. Pontis A, et al. Adenomyosis: a systematic review of medical treatment. Gynecol Endocrinol. 2016;32(9):696–700.
6. Marnach ML, Laughlin-Tommaso SK. Evaluation and management of abnormal uterine bleeding. Mayo Clinic Proc. 2019. Elsevier;94(2):326–35.
7. Shaaban OM, et al. Levonorgestrel-releasing intrauterine system versus a low-dose combined oral contraceptive for treatment of adenomyotic uteri: a randomized clinical trial. Contraception. 2015;92(4):301–7.
8. Li L, et al. A prospective cohort study on effects of levonorgestrel-releasing intrauterine system for adenomyosis with severe dysmenorrhea. Zhonghua Fu Chan Ke Za Zhi. 2016;51(5):345–51.
9. Andersson K, Odlind V, Rybo G. Levonorgestrel-releasing and copper-releasing (Nova T) IUDs during five years of use: a randomized comparative trial. Contraception. 1994;49(1):56–72.
10. Backman T, et al. Advance information improves user satisfaction with the levonorgestrel intrauterine system. Obstet Gynecol. 2002;99(4):608–13.
11. Agostinho L, et al. MRI for adenomyosis: a pictorial review. Insights Imaging. 2017;8(6):549–56.
12. Kishi Y, et al. Four subtypes of adenomyosis assessed by magnetic resonance imaging and their specification. Am J Obstet Gynecol. 2012;207(2):114.e1–7.
13. Bazot M, Daraï E. Role of transvaginal sonography and magnetic resonance imaging in the diagnosis of uterine adenomyosis. Fertil Steril. 2018;109(3):389–97.
14. Lazzeri L, et al. A sonographic classification of adenomyosis: interobserver reproducibility in the evaluation of type and degree of the myometrial involvement. Fertil Steril. 2018;110(6):1154–1161.e3.
15. Sun Y, et al. Prevalence of abnormal uterine bleeding according to new International Federation of Gynecology and Obstetrics classification in Chinese women of reproductive age: a cross-sectional study. Medicine. 2018;97(31):e11457.
16. Shazly SA, et al. Intraoperative predictors of long-term outcomes after radiofrequency endometrial ablation. J Minim Invasive Gynecol. 2016;23(4):582–9.
17. Philip C-A, et al. Evaluation of NovaSure® global endometrial ablation in symptomatic adenomyosis: a longitudinal study with a 36 month follow-up. Eur J Obstet Gynecol Reprodu Biol. 2018;227:46–51.
18. Taran F, Stewart EA, Brucker S. Adenomyosis: epidemiology, risk factors, clinical phenotype and surgical and interventional alternatives to hysterectomy. Geburtshilfe Frauenheilkd. 2013;73(09):924–31.
19. Cheung VY. Current status of high-intensity focused ultrasound for the management of uterine adenomyosis. Ultrasonography. 2017;36(2):95.
20. Benetti-Pinto CL, et al. Pharmacological treatment for symptomatic Adenomyosis: a systematic review. Revista Brasileira de Ginecologia e Obstetrícia/RBGO Gynecology and Obstetrics. 2019;41(09):564–74.
21. Osuga Y, Fujimoto-Okabe H, Hagino A. Evaluation of the efficacy and safety of dienogest in the treatment of painful symptoms in patients with adenomyosis: a randomized, double-blind, multicenter, placebo-controlled study. Fertil Steril. 2017;108(4):673–8.
22. Osuga Y, Watanabe M, Hagino A. Long-term use of dienogest in the treatment of painful symptoms in adenomyosis. J Obstet Gynaecol Res. 2017;43(9):1441–8.
23. Neriishi K, et al. Long-term dienogest administration in patients with symptomatic adenomyosis. J Obstet Gynaecol Res. 2018;44(8):1439–44.
24. Matsushima T, et al. Recurrence of uterine adenomyosis after administration of gonadotropin-releasing hormone agonist and the efficacy of dienogest. Gynecol Endocrinol. 2019;22:1–4.
25. Ota K, et al. Combination of microwave endometrial ablation and postoperative dienogest administration is effective for treating symptomatic adenomyosis. J Obstet Gynaecol Res. 2018;44(9):1787–92.

Adenomyosis and Infertility

Guoyun Wang

Uterine adenomyosis is a benign gynecological disease that affects women's fertility and quality of life. Infertility, miscarriage, and obstetric complications are prominent problems, which are difficult and hot spots in its research and treatment. There is an increasing evidence that adenomyosis is associated with infertility and reproductive failure [1–4]. A recent cross-sectional study of infertile women found that the incidence of adenomyosis was 29.7% in women over 40 years of age and 22% under 40 years of age. Furthermore, among people with repeated miscarriages and previous assisted reproductive technology (ART) failures, this proportion increased to 38.2% [5].

7.1 Factors Influencing Fertility in Adenomyosis

Infertility is the main clinical symptom in patients with adenomyosis. The possible mechanisms of infertility caused by adenomyosis are as follows: (a) Abnormal anatomical structure: adenomyosis often has an abnormal uterine cavity morphology, which may obstruct the fallopian tube opening, interfere with sperm transport and embryo implantation, or increased uterine volume compressing the surrounding fallopian tubes and ovaries, affecting the peristalsis of the fallopian tube and the function of collecting eggs in the pelvis, and thus affects the fertilization [6]. (b) The thickness of the endometrial-myometrial interface (EMI), or called junctional zone (JZ), increases, causing dysfunctional uterine peristalsis. Furthermore, the ultra-structure changes of the myometrium make the muscle cells contract abnormally, causing loss of rhythm of uterine contraction, leading to impaired sperm transport and affecting fertilization and embryo implantation [7]. (c) Adenomyosis is an

G. Wang (✉)
Department of Obstetrics and Gynecology, Qilu Hospital of Shandong University, Jinan, Shandong, China
e-mail: wangguoy@sdu.edu.cn

© The Author(s), under exclusive license to Springer Nature Singapore Pte Ltd. 2021
M. Xue et al. (eds.), *Adenomyosis*, https://doi.org/10.1007/978-981-33-4095-4_7

inflammatory disease. Studies have found that patients with adenomyosis often have endometrial lesions, mainly endometrial polyps and endometritis. Endometrial polyps can cause disorders of embryo implantation, and the local inflammatory cells and factors in endometritis increase, killing and phagocytizing sperm interfering with the histocompatibility of embryos and the endometrium [8, 9]. (d) Endometrial dysfunction in patients with adenomyosis, including abnormalities in sex hormone synthesis and conduction pathways, decreased expression of implantation markers, reduced expression of adhesion molecules, changes in embryonic developmental genes (such as HOXA 10), increased release of free radicals, and endometrial vascularization disorders, etc., leading to abnormal embryo implantation and early abortion [10]. (e) Serum prolactin (PRL) levels in patients with adenomyosis are significantly higher than those in the control group. High levels of PRL can inhibit the secretion of follicle-stimulating hormone (FSH) and luteinizing hormone (LH), thereby affecting the function of the corpus luteum. High levels of PRL in the follicular phase can inhibit the synthesis and secretion of sex hormones, leading to disorders of follicular development, maturation, and ovulation. At the same time, the positive rate of PRL receptors in adenomyosis lesions is significantly increased, leading to an imbalance of sex hormones, which may lead to infertility [11].

7.2   Pregnancy Outcomes in Adenomyosis

Adenomyosis not only causes infertility but also affects pregnancy outcomes. Studies have found an increased risk of premature rupture of membranes and preterm birth in patients with adenomyosis [12]. The incidence of cesarean section, small-for-gestational age, postpartum hemorrhage, and fetal malpresentation in patients with adenomyosis also increased [13]. A current case-control study found that the incidence of second-trimester miscarriage, preeclampsia, and placental abnormalities in patients with adenomyosis also increased significantly [14]. Different types of adenomyosis have different effects on pregnancy outcomes. The incidence of pregnancy-induced hypertension and uterine infections in diffuse adenomyosis patients is higher than localized, and the incidence of cervical insufficiency is also increased [15]. These have led to an increased incidence of abortion, premature labor, and obstetric complications in patients with adenomyosis. These factors may end with secondary infertility in patients with adenomyosis.

7.3   Adenomyosis with Endometriosis

The influence of ultrasound classification of adenomyosis on infertility is also different. A prospective study by Exacoustos et al. 2019 [16] showed that localized lesions had a higher incidence of infertility than diffuse lesions, and that the prevalence of abortions in localized lesions involving the JZ was higher than that of diffuse lesions. Adenomyosis is often associated with endometriosis, especially in infertile patients, and the proportion can be as high as 79% [17]. Pelvic endometriosis can cause dense adhesions of the ovary and fallopian tubes, leading to distortion of the fallopian tubes. In severe cases, the tubal obstruction can occur. When the ovarian endometriotic cyst ruptures, it can cause widespread inflammation, leading to omental adhesions and wrapping affecting the peristalsis of the fallopian tubes. The adhesion and encapsulation of the ovary affect the oocyte discharge. If the endometriosis destroys the ovarian parenchyma, it will affect egg production. Uterine adhesion makes it difficult for sperms to enter the uterine cavity and can also cause infertility. Besides, endometriotic lesions, involving the fallopian tube, can cause tubal obstruction, thereby affecting its function [18]. Patients with endometriosis often have neuroendocrine dysfunction, which leads to poor follicular development, impaired LH peak formation, or insensitivity of follicles to LH, or mechanical factors, such as adhesions, leading to luteinized unruptured follicle syndrome (LUFS), and endometriosis with LUFS accounts for about 18–79%. Endometriosis is also often associated with luteal dysfunction, with an incidence of about 25–45%. Luteal dysfunction is one of the causes of infertility in patients with adenomyosis and endometriosis. The peritoneal fluid of patients with endometriosis contains a large number of activated immune cells and cytokines, which can swallow sperm, affect sperm activity, hinder fertilization, and have apparent toxic effects on embryos, affecting early embryo development and implantation, causing infertility and early abortion. The peritoneal fluid of patients with endometriosis contains high concentrations of prostaglandin (PG). PG can cause abnormal uterine contractions and tubal peristalsis, so that by the time the zygotes reach the uterine cavity, it is not synchronized with the development of the endometrium and affect the implantation of the fertilized eggs, causing early abortion [19].

References

1. Younes G, Tulandi T. Effects of adenomyosis on in vitro fertilization treatment outcomes: a meta-analysis. Fertil Steril. 2017;108:483–490.e3.
2. Tomassetti C, et al. Adenomyosis and subfertility: evidence of association and causation. Semin Reprod Med. 2013;31(2):101–8.
3. Benagiano, Adenomyosis and infertility. Reproductive Biomedicine Online.
4. Vercellini P, et al. Uterine adenomyosis and in vitro fertilization outcome: a systematic review and meta-analysis. Hum Reprod. 2014;29(5):964–77.
5. Garcia-Velasco JA. Adenomyosis in infertile women: prevalence and the role of 3D ultrasound as a marker of severity of the disease. Reprod Biol Endocrinol. 2016;14(1):60.
6. Harada T, et al. The Impact of Adenomyosis on Women's fertility. Obstet Gynecol Surv. 2016;71(9):557–68.
7. Habiba MA. Uterine adenomyosis is associated with ultrastructural features of altered contractility in the inner myometrium. Fertil Steril. 2009;93(7):P2130–6.
8. Mall G. The pathophysiology of endometriosis and adenomyosis: tissue injury and repair. Arch Gynecol Obstet. 2009;280(4):529–38.
9. Lieng M, Istre O, Qvigstad E. Treatment of endometrial polyps: a systematic review. J Minim Invasive Gynecol. 2010;89(8):992–1002.
10. Petraglia F. Pathogenesis of adenomyosis: an update on molecular mechanisms. Reprod Biomed Online. 2017; 35(5):592–601. http://www.rbmojournal.com/article/S1472648317302961/pdf.

11. Jiang Y, et al. Decreased expression of NR4A nuclear receptors in adenomyosis impairs endo-metrial decidualization. Mhr: Basic Sci Reprod Med. 2016;22(9):655–68.
12. Hsu WL. Adenomyosis and risk of preterm delivery. BJOG Int J Obstet Gynaecol. 2007;114(2):165–9.
13. Mochimaru A, et al. Adverse pregnancy outcomes associated with adenomyosis with uterine enlargement. J Obstet Gynaecol Res. 2015;41(4):529–33.
14. Hashimoto A, Iriyama T, Sayama S Fujii T et al. Adenomyosis and adverse perinatal out-comes: increased risk of second trimester miscarriage, preeclampsia, and placental malposi-tion. J Matern Fetal Neonatal Med, 2018, 31p 1–6.
15. Tamura H, Maekawa R, Sugino N. Complications and outcomes of pregnant women with adenomyosis in Japan. Fertil Steril. 2018;110(4):e389–90.
16. Exacoustos C, et al. New sonographic classification of adenomyosis: do type and degree of ade-nomyosis correlate to severity of symptoms? J Minim Invasive Gynecol. 2019;27(6):1308–15.
17. Kunz G, et al. Adenomyosis in endometriosis—prevalence and impact on fertility. Evidence from magnetic resonance imaging. Hum Reprod. 2005;20(8):2309–16.
18. Lisa J, Rubin I, Trinidad S. Further observations on ectopic endometrium of the fallopian tube. Surg Gynecol Obstet. 1956;103(4):469.
19. Na Y-J, et al. Effects of peritoneal fluid from endometriosis patients on the release of vascular endothelial growth factor by neutrophils and monocytes. Hum Reprod. 2006;21(7):1846–55.

Ultrasound Manifestation and Classification of Adenomyosis

8

Qing Dai and Jinhua Leng

At present, the commonly used diagnostic imaging examinations of adenomyosis are MRI and ultrasound. Ultrasound imaging is the first-line imaging method of choice for adenomyosis, because its practice is simple, easily repeatable, low cost, and with clear images and has no contraindications. Therefore ultrasound has been widely used in the diagnosis, classification, and follow-up observation of drugs and surgery after adenomyosis. The literature on ultrasound diagnosis of adenomyosis started in the 1980s. Transabdominal ultrasound was used to diagnose adenomyosis based on the sonographic uterine enlargement and asymmetric thickening of the anterior or/and posterior wall of the myometrium [1]. With the increasing use of transvaginal ultrasound (TVUS) after the 1990s, the high resolution of TVUS can give more detailed and comprehensive uterine features to diagnose adenomyosis with great certainty. Also, ultrasound examination has the advantages of simplicity, no radiation, easy repeatability, and low cost. At present, TVUS has been widely used in clinical practice and became the first and irreplaceable imaging examination for adenomyosis [2]. This chapter describes the ultrasound technology, imaging appearances, classification, differential diagnosis of adenomyosis, and advances in ultrasound imaging of adenomyosis.

8.1 Ultrasound Technology

Ultrasound for adenomyosis can be divided into different approaches: (1) transabdominal ultrasound, (2) transvaginal ultrasound, and (3) transrectal ultrasound.

Q. Dai (✉) · J. Leng
Department of Obstetrics and Gynecology, Peking Union Medical College Hospital, Beijing, China

© The Author(s), under exclusive license to Springer Nature Singapore Pte Ltd. 2021
M. Xue et al. (eds.), *Adenomyosis*, https://doi.org/10.1007/978-981-33-4095-4_8

8.1.1 Transabdominal Ultrasound

Subjects need to drink 500–1000 ml of water before the examination to fill the bladder. The ultrasound probe is a convex array probe, and the center frequency of the probe is 3.5 MHz. During the scan, the lower abdomen is exposed first, and an appropriate amount of coupling materials (usually ultrasound gel) is applied onto the abdomen. The probe is directly put on the skin of the abdominal wall for scanning. First, a longitudinal view of the uterus is scanned (Figure 8.1), and the uterine length, anteroposterior diameter, and endometrial thickness are measured. Then rotate the probe 90° for cross-section scan and measure the transverse uterine diameter; carefully observe any uterine lesions and both the adnexal areas. During the scanning, the probe is flexibly moved according to the lesions or the area of interest, with the scanning direction and angle changed to obtain the best image of the lesions, if any.

Transabdominal ultrasound scans have a wide range, flexible planes, and free scan angles and can display the full picture of the larger uterus. It is one of the commonly used ultrasound examination methods, but it is susceptible to factors, such as abdominal wall thickness, bladder filling degree, and intestinal flatulence.

8.1.2 Transvaginal Ultrasound

TVUS is ultrasonography with an ultrasound probe inserted into the vagina. It is one of the most commonly used ultrasound methods in gynecology. Subjects need to empty the bladder before the test. The examiner prepared a vaginal probe with a covering condom. For patients with vaginal bleeding, when TVUS is indeed necessary for diagnosis, the examiner should use a sterile condom. The subject routinely lays in a lithotomy position. If necessary, use a pillow to raise the hips or ask the examinee to place their hands under the hips to raise it. The ultrasound probe is for transvaginal use with a center frequency of 7.5 MHz.

Fig. 8.1 Transabdominal ultrasound showing a normal longitudinal view of the uterus, *BL* bladder, *UT* uterus

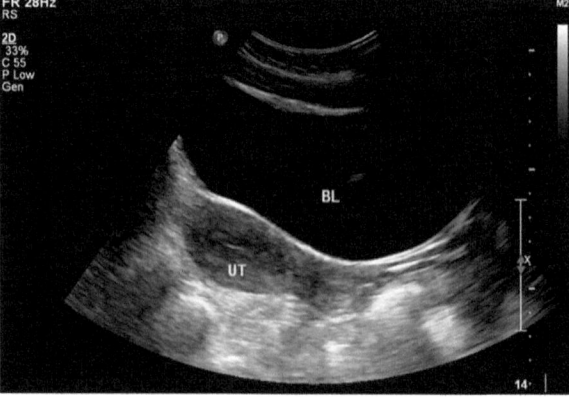

During the scan, the longitudinal, transverse, and oblique planes of the pelvic structure are scanned using basic scanning techniques, such as rotation, tilt, and pumping. Measure the longitudinal uterine length, anterior and posterior wall diameters, and endometrial thickness on the longitudinal section of the uterus (Fig. 8.2); rotate the probe 90° to measure the transverse width of the uterus on the cross-section. Then carefully examine the uterus for any lesions and move the probe to the left or right side of the uterus to scan the left and right adnexal areas, including the bilateral ovaries and surrounding adnexa. During the scanning process, the probe should be flexibly moved, according to the lesion or the area of interest, and the scanning direction and angle should be changed to perform multi-section scanning to obtain the best image of any uterine lesion.

Due to the high frequency of transvaginal probe and its proximity to the pelvic organs and excellent image resolution, it can better display the structural characteristics and blood flow of uterine, ovarian, and pelvic masses and is not affected by bowel gas interference and abdominal wall sound attenuation. It is suitable for patients who can undergo a transvaginal examination. TVUS is superior to transabdominal ultrasound in the detailed observation of uterine lesions. However, although the transvaginal probe has a high frequency, its penetrating power is limited, and it is difficult to comprehensively observe a larger uterus, which needs to combine with a transabdominal ultrasound examination. TVUS cannot be performed on a virgin and vagina with congenital deformities, vaginal infection, and severe senile vaginal atrophy with stenosis.

8.1.3   Transrectal Ultrasound

Transrectal ultrasound is an approach to place an intraluminal probe in the rectum for an ultrasound examination. It is used for patients whose transabdominal ultrasound images are not clear but who cannot have a TVUS examination. Subjects need to empty the bowel and bladder before the transrectal examination. Generally, take laxatives the night before the examination and with an empty stomach on the

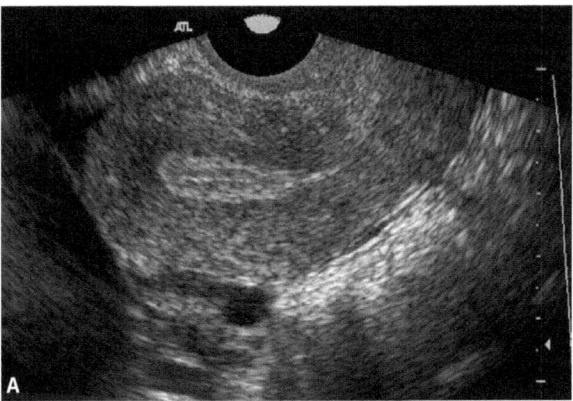

Fig. 8.2 TVUS shows a normal longitudinal section of the uterus

morning of the test. The subject takes a left lateral position with the left leg straight and the right leg flexed. Sometimes a supine lithotomy position can also be used. A transrectal probe is used, which can be the same probe used as the transvaginal probe.

After the probe is mounted with a latex condom, an appropriate amount of coupling agent should be added to the condom as a lubricant to facilitate the placement of the probe into the rectum. The scanning method and observation sequence are the same as those of transvaginal scanning.

8.2 Comparison of Transvaginal Ultrasound and Magnetic Resonance Imaging

The advantages of TVUS over magnetic resonance imaging (MRI) are mainly its universal applicability, economy, and easy repeatability. MRI uses quantifiable and specific diagnostic criteria to make the imaging diagnosis of adenomyosis more reliable; especially MRI can better show the endometrial-myometrial junctional zone (JZ). The JZ at T2W imaging showed that focal or diffuse thickening of the uterine wall is closely associated with adenomyosis [3]. Although the ultrasound does not show the JZ as distinctly as MRI, the ultrasound image can clearly show a series of sonographic features corresponding to the pathological changes of adenomyosis. It can be widely practiced in general medical office environments, and it is relatively cheap and well-tolerated and has no preparation required and no contraindications, particularly highly accurate in the hands of ultrasound experts. Therefore it becomes the preferred imaging examination for adenomyosis [4].

Compared with TVUS, the diagnostic accuracy of MRI was slightly higher in earlier studies. However, in recent years, with the continuous improvement of ultrasound technology and diagnostic level, the diagnostic accuracy of ultrasound for adenomyosis has been similar to that of MRI. The literature reported that both TVUS and MRI have high accuracy in the diagnosis of adenomyosis. Data from one study showed that the overall sensitivity of TVUS is 72% (95% CI 65–79%), and the specificity is 81% (95% CI 77–85%), while the overall sensitivity of MRI is 77% (95% CI 67–85%), and the specificity is 89% (95% CI 84–92%) [5]. Similar data from another study showed that TVUS had a sensitivity and specificity of 84% and 91.9%, respectively, while that of MRI were 88% and 94.6%, respectively. The accuracy rates of TVUS and MRI were 87.4% and 90.8% [4]. Therefore, the accuracy of TVUS and MRI in diagnosing adenomyosis is similar. Furthermore, the application of three-dimensional (3D) TVUS significantly improves the ability of ultrasound to display the uterine JZ and the diagnosis of adenomyosis.

8.3 Ultrasound Findings Reflect Histopathological Features

Ultrasound appearance of adenomyosis includes abnormal enlargement of the uterus, changes in the myometrial echogenicity, changes in the endometrial-myometrial JZ (changes in JZ), and abnormal uterine activity.

The ultrasound appearance of adenomyosis is based on its pathological changes. Histopathologically, adenomyosis is the invasion of the endometrial glands and stroma into the myometrium. Periodic bleeding occurs with the menstrual cycle, forming microcystic lesions, accompanied by reactive hyperplasia and hypertrophy of surrounding muscle fibers in the myometrium, forming a thickened fibrous muscular layer; the usual boundary between the endometrium and the muscular layer is destroyed, and the endometrium invades the inner muscle layer. The endometrium invades more than 2.5 mm to the underlying muscle layer or up to more than 25% of the myometrial thickness, forming adenomyosis.

Ultrasound images can clearly show the sonographic features that correspond to the pathological changes of adenomyosis and reflect the histological features [6], such as endometrial and myometrial injury leads to the growth of endometrial glands and stromal into the myometrium. Thus it gives rise to the ultrasound appearance of linear and bud-like hyperechoic islands below the endometrium.

According to the growth characteristics of adenomyosis, it can be divided into focal adenomyosis and diffuse adenomyosis. Histologically, if the endometrial glands and interstitials appear as a nodule, with its periphery surrounded by normal myometrium, this is a focal type of adenomyosis. When the endometrial glands in the myometrium are diffusely distributed, it is called diffuse adenomyosis. Adenomyoma is a subgroup of focal adenomyosis surrounded by a thick layer of myometrium [7].

8.4 Ultrasound Features of Adenomyosis

The main ultrasound features of adenomyosis include uterine spheroid enlargement, asymmetry thickening of the anterior or posterior myometrium of the uterus, myometrial heterogeneity, small cysts, and microcysts in the affected muscular layer. Besides, there may be fan-shaped sound shadows, moderate-high echogenic lines (linear stripes) or island nodules under the endometrium, unclear JZ, etc. Also, the color Doppler flow image shows blood flow signals in the adenomyosis lesion of the myometrium. Increased blood flow presents as penetrating vascularity. Whether it is diffuse adenomyosis or focal or adenomyoma, the heterogeneity in the lesion, rough, small cystic, or microcystic structures and the increase in color doppler flow imaging (CDFI) blood flow signals are common ultrasound manifestations of adenomyosis [6–12].

8.4.1 The Uterus Is Enlarged, with the Asymmetry of the Anterior and Posterior Walls of the Uterus

In diffuse adenomyosis, uterine enlargement is often manifested as a spherical enlargement (Figure 8.3a, b) with the enlargement of the entire uterine body, excluding the cervix. A normal uterus is inverted pear-shaped. When spherical, it shows that the anterior and posterior diameters increase significantly, there is no convex mass, and the uterine outline is not deformed. Even focal adenomyomas usually do not present with abnormal uterine contours like leiomyoma. Of course, the uterus with mild adenomyosis can be normal in size.

Myometrial thickening can be focal or diffuse. The former is a manifestation of focal adenomyosis. In diffuse adenomyosis, only a few cases show an increase in the anterior and posterior wall of the uterus and the fundus of the uterus (Fig. 8.4). The thickening of the anterior and posterior walls is asymmetric. Adenomyosis most often affects the uterine fundus and posterior wall area, less to the anterior wall, and rarely the uterine horn or the cervix. Therefore, the asymmetric thickening of the anterior and posterior uterine muscle layers is a common ultrasound manifestation of diffuse adenomyosis, and the posterior uterine wall and uterine fundal thickening are the most common (Fig. 8.5). Only a few manifest as anterior wall

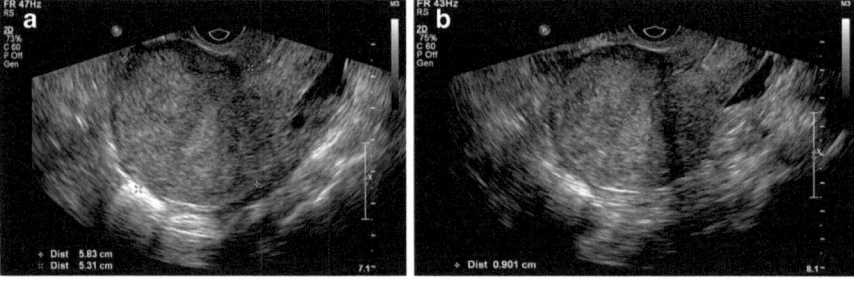

Fig. 8.3 (a and b): TVUS images, all of which are longitudinal sections of the uterus, and the uterus is spherically enlarged. (a) shows the measurement of the size of the uterus. (b) shows the measurement of the endometrium

Fig. 8.4 Transabdominal ultrasound image of diffuse adenomyosis, showing that the uterine body is diffusely and uniformly enlarged, that is, the uterine fundus, anterior wall, and posterior wall are all enlarged; the cervix is normal size

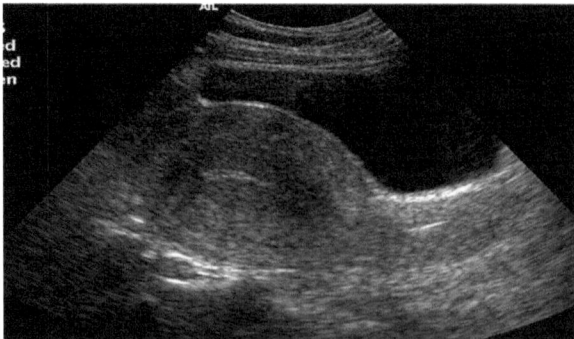

thickening (Fig. 8.6), and the majority of cases have a normal cervix, resulting in a significantly disproportionate size of the uterine body and the cervix.

In focal adenomyosis, the uterine myometrium is focally thickened and behaves similarly to uterine fibroids, but the boundary of the adenomyosis lesion is unclear (Figure 8.7a and b). Internal echo has the characteristics of adenomyosis, such as heterogeneity, rough, fan-shaped sound shadow, small cysts or microcysts, etc.; some focal lesions may have an easily distinguished boundary, and they are called adenomyoma (Fig. 8.8), but the border of adenomyoma is still less precise compared with that of uterine fibroid.

Fig. 8.5 TVUS image of diffuse adenomyosis, showing increased asymmetry of the anterior and posterior wall of the uterus. The uterus shows mainly the thickness of the posterior wall. The thickness of the posterior wall is 2.89 cm, while the anterior wall is only 0.99 cm

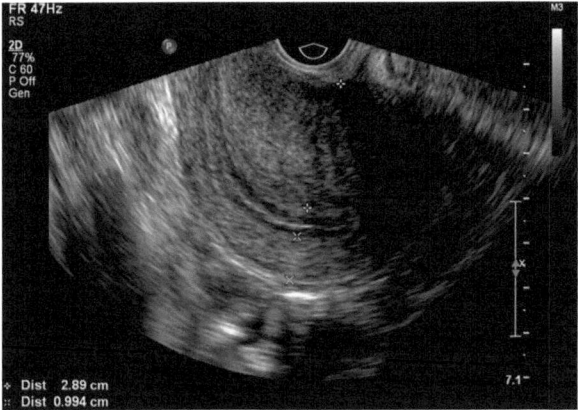

Fig. 8.6 TVUS image of diffuse adenomyosis showing increased asymmetry of the anterior and posterior wall of the uterus, the uterus is anteverted; the anterior wall of the uterus has a thickness of 3.5 cm and the posterior wall 0.9 cm

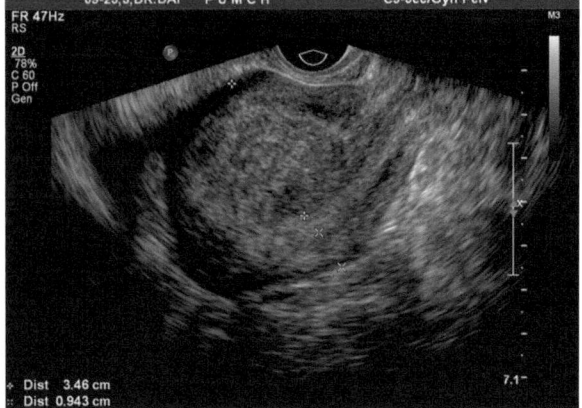

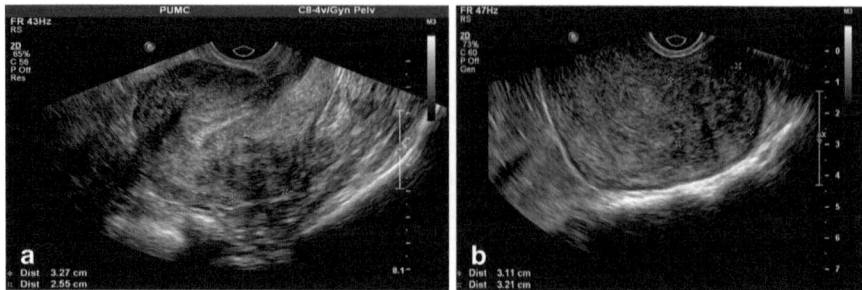

Fig. 8.7 (**a**) TVUS image of focal adenomyosis. The uterus is anteverted, showing a focal enlargement of the posterior wall of the uterus, the range of the lesion is 3.3 cm × 2.6 cm, the boundary of adenomyoma is unclear, and the internal echo is heterogeneous with partial pencil-like sound shadow (**b**) TVUS image of focal adenomyosis. The uterus is retroverted, showing a focal increase in the posterior wall of the uterus near the fundus of the uterus. The size of the lesion is 3.2 cm × 3.1 cm. It is difficult to distinguish a clear border of the entire lesion

Fig. 8.8 Transabdominal ultrasound image of focal adenomyoma. The uterus is anteverted, showing that the posterior wall of the uterus is focally enlarged, and the boundary of the lesion is unclear. The border of the lesion can still be distinguished, because it protrudes towards the surface of the uterus. There are heterogeneous inside the lesion

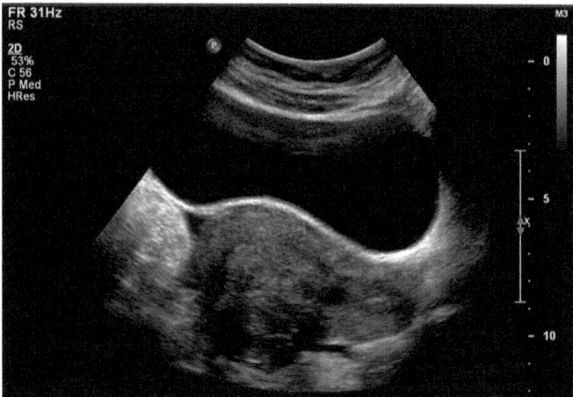

8.4.2 Heterogeneity of the Myometrium

Regardless of diffuse or focal adenomyosis, the heterogeneity of the affected myometrium is the most common ultrasound manifestation of adenomyosis [13]. The unevenness is mainly due to the echogenic changes of the uterine myometrium and low echo alternating with hyperechoic stripes or nodules; the arrangement is disordered, making the uterine texture significantly heterogeneous and rough (Figure 8.9a, b), similar to the manifestation of liver cirrhosis in end-stage liver disease. Meanwhile, multiple linear sound shadows also cause heterogeneity. The degree of echo unevenness also reflects the severity of adenomyosis to a certain extent.

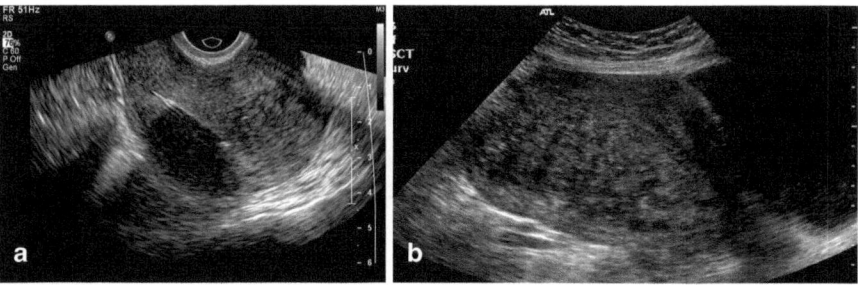

Fig. 8.9 (**a**) TVUS image of adenomyosis. The uterus is retroverted. The picture shows the echotexture of the posterior uterine muscle layer changes, with uneven echo and thicken wall; meanwhile, the intrauterine cavity shows the high echoes of the Mirena IUCD, and the sound shadow behind it. The echoes of the myometrium of the anterior wall of the uterus are not seen clearly (**b**) Transabdominal ultrasound image of adenomyosis. The uterus is anteverted; the picture shows that the echo of the posterior wall of the uterus is obviously uneven and rough, and the hypoechoic stripes and hyperechoic stripes or nodules alternately exist. The arrangement is disordered, and the posterior wall is significantly thicker than the anterior wall

8.4.3 Small Cysts or Microcysts in the Affected Myometrium

Cyclic bleeding of the ectopic endometrial glands in the myometrium can lead to the formation of small cysts or microcysts in the myometrium. Cysts are usually 1–5 mm in diameter and are generally in the form of non-echoic areas (Figure 8.10a, b, and c). Because the fluid in the sac is old blood, small cysts can also appear as hypoechoic cysts. By reducing the field of view and enlarging the ultrasound image, the display effect of these cysts can be improved. Due to the active endometrial tissue and inflammatory response around the cyst, there is a hyperechoic rim around the cyst, appearing like a thick cyst wall (Fig. 8.11).

Small cysts in the myometrium are very specific ultrasound features of adenomyosis. As early as the beginning of this century, research by Bazot et al. [13] showed that small uterine myometrial cysts are the most sensitive and specific criteria for ultrasound diagnosis of adenomyosis. More recent studies [14] have shown that the most specific ultrasound feature of TVUS for the diagnosis of adenomyosis is myometrial cysts (98% specificity), and the most sensitive ultrasound feature is the heterogeneity of the myometrium (88% sensitivity). Besides, the linear echoes perpendicular to the endometrium under the intima can be seen filled with liquid and present as a linear anechoic zone [7].

8.4.4 Fan-Shaped Sound Shadow in the Uterus

The other characteristic ultrasound features, which is as important as the myometrial heterogeneity, is a fan-shaped sound shadow caused by the changes of the texture of the uterine myometrium, also known as the shutter sign, multiple linear or pencil-shaped sound shadow [7]. In adenomyosis, the hyperechoic and hypoechoic

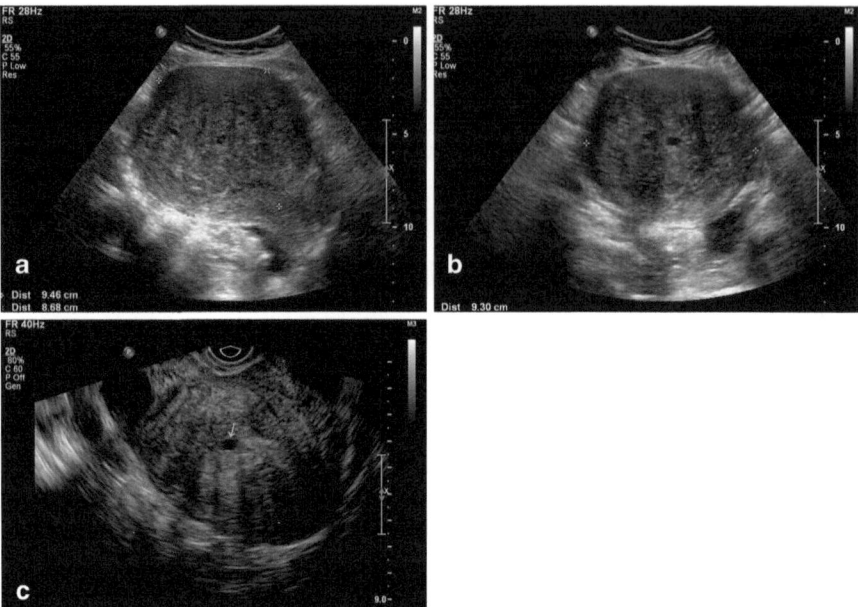

Fig. 8.10 (**a** and **b**) Transabdominal ultrasound images of diffuse adenomyosis, the uterus is ante-verted, which shows that the anterior uterine muscle layer is significantly thickened, and the echo is heterogeneous. Multiple small anechoic areas scattered in the lesion are visible. (**c**) TVUS image of adenomyosis. The uterus is anteverted. It shows that the anterior wall of the uterus is thickened, and the echo is uneven. Several small anechoic areas (pointed by arrows) are visible

Fig. 8.11 TVUS image of adenomyosis. The uterus is anteverted, showing that the anterior wall of the uterus is thickened, and the echo is significantly uneven. There are several small anechoic areas and hyperechoic rim around the anechoic area

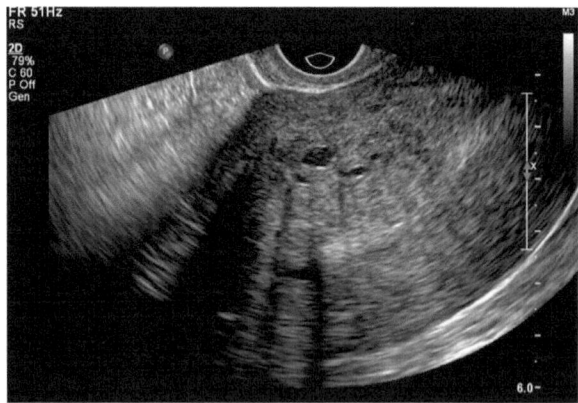

areas appear alternately and disorderly in the uterine myometrium. The normal myometrial echotexture disappears, and the echo becomes heterogeneous and rough. Many vertical and thin radially fan-shaped sound shadows (Figure 8.12a-c) are identified.

Although leiomyomas can have fan-shaped sound shadows like adenomyosis, the sound shadows of uterine fibroids are more likely to be caused by dense calcification or by attenuation of fibrous components or lateral sound shadows of the cystic areas. The width of the sound shadow varies, as shown in Fig. 8.13. A large leiomyoma can sometimes completely obscure the ultrasound manifestations of adenomyosis, at which point MRI is needed to help determine the presence of adenomyosis.

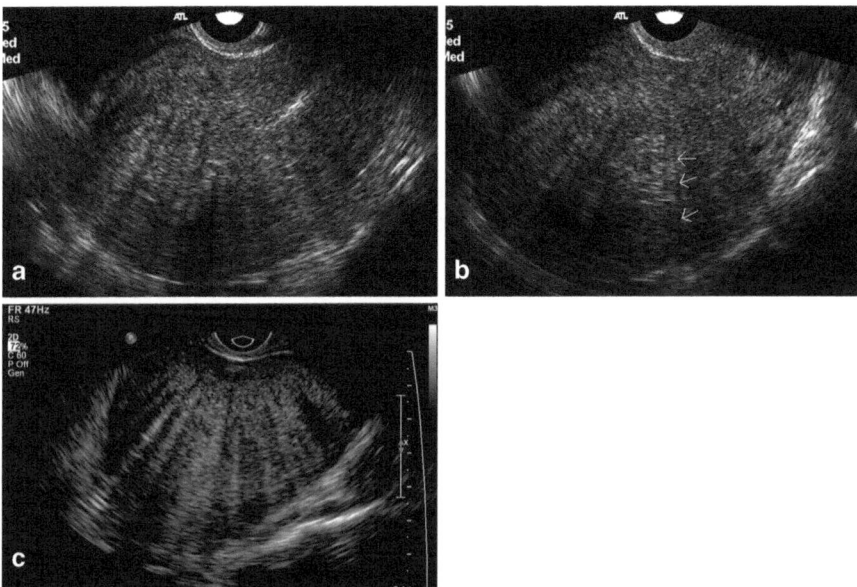

Fig. 8.12 (**a-c**): TVUS images of adenomyosis show that in addition to the enlargement of the uterus and uneven echos of the uterine myometrium, fan-shaped sound shadows can be seen in the uterus and appear as straight and thin streaks or pencils-like sound shadows. These sound shadows are arranged in a fan-shaped or jalousie-like arrangement

Fig. 8.13 TVUS image of uterine fibroids, showing that the acoustic shadow of uterine fibroids is different from that of adenomyosis. The fibroid image shows a well-defined hypoechoic lesion in the uterus, sometimes with the hyperechoic lesion, and a wide range of sound shadows behind it

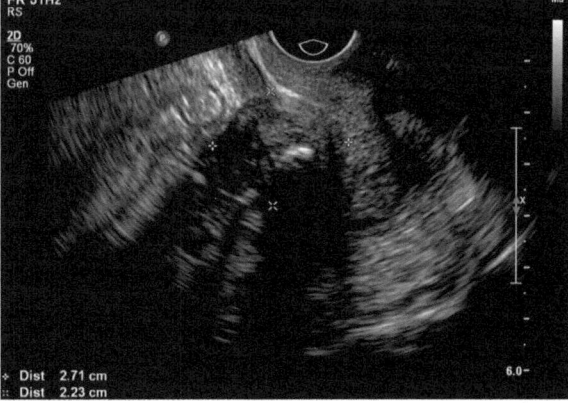

8.4.5 Linear, bud, or Island-like Hyperechoic Nodules under the Endometrium

In adenomyosis, the endometrial-myometrial demarcation is unclear (Figure 8.14a), or hyperechoic linear, bud-like echo stripes, or island nodules can be seen in the region of the endometrial zone. Uterine adenomyosis is where the glands and stroma of the endometrium invade the myometrium in an "inside-out" order. The above manifestations represent the endometrial tissue extending directly into the myometrium, with linear stripes or island nodules extend into the muscular layer from the endometrial boundary (Figure 8.14b). The linear endometrial streaks are the most special ultrasound feature of adenomyosis and have high diagnostic accuracy [7].

8.4.6 The Endometrial-Myometrial Junctional Zone (JZ) Is Thickened, Irregular, Interrupted or Difficult to Distinguish

The endometrial-myometrial JZ is a muscle layer structure, which is a transitional region between the endometrium and the muscle layer. It consists of longitudinal and circular, tightly arranged smooth muscle fibers. The blurred boundary of the endometrial-myometrial boundary in the adenomyosis is mainly due to changes in the uterine JZ caused by the endometrial invasion. MRI has a typical feature for the thickening of the JZ, but it is still difficult to measure the JZ accurately on ultrasound. However, in the recent 10 years, with 3D ultrasound technology and volume contrast imaging (VCI) and other new ultrasound technologies increasingly applied in clinical practice, ultrasound has been able to evaluate the uterine JZ reliably [11]. Kepkep et al. 2007 [12] reported that 3D TVUS makes the display of JZ clearer, and the unclear boundary of JZ has a high specificity (82%) for the diagnosis of adenomyosis. Exacoustos et al. 2011 [14] reported that on 3D

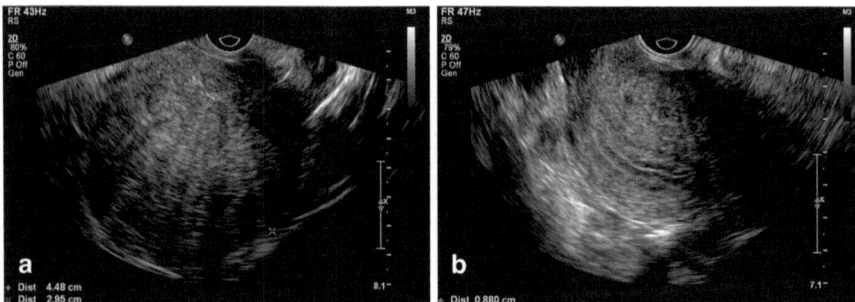

Fig. 8.14 (**a** and **b**) TVUS images of adenomyosis. (**a**) presents an anteverted uterus. The image shows diffuse adenomyosis; the anteroposterior walls are thickened, the echoes are significantly uneven, the fan-shaped sound shadow, and the endometrial-myometrial boundary is unclear, making it difficult to distinguish the endometrial border. (**b**) presents a posterior uterus, and the image shows linear streaks visible under the endometrium

TVUS, the maximum thickness of the JZ (JZ max) $\geq$ 8 mm or the difference between the maximum and minimum JZ thickness (JZ diff) $\geq$ 4 mm might be possibly adenomyosis.

8.4.7 Increased Blood Flow Signal in the Lesion, with Penetrating Vascular Feature

In adenomyosis, due to myofibrosis and hypertrophy of the uterine myometrium, blood vessels in the uterine myometrium have also generally increased. CDFI showed increased blood flow signals in the uterine myometrial area (Figure 8.15a, b, c, and d); the blood flow presents as a penetrating blood flow (straight blood vessels are present), and more tortuous blood vessels pass through the affected myometrium [8]. This feature is also seen in angiography.

The area of increased blood flow signals in the myometrium can reflect the extent and distribution of adenomyosis. At the same time, the CDFI manifestations of adenomyosis can also help distinguish between adenomyosis and uterine fibroids [15].

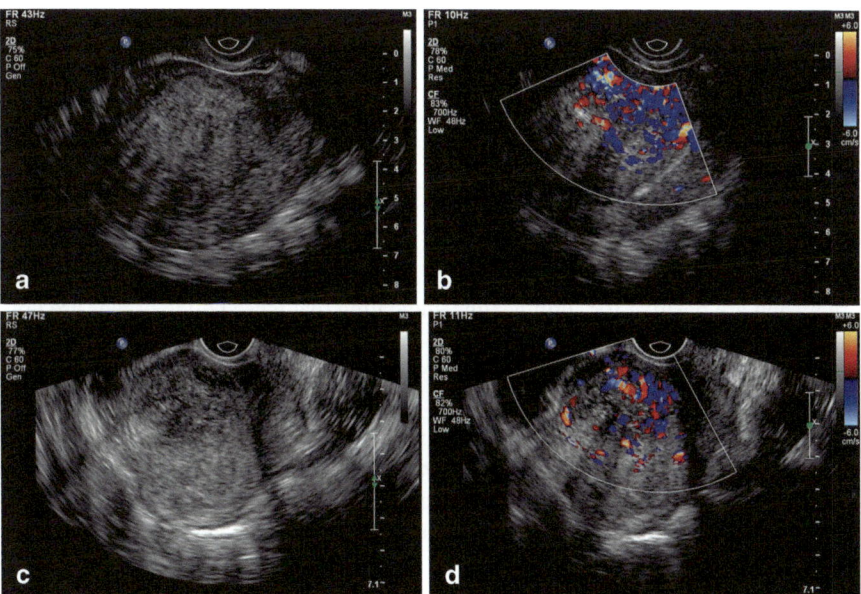

Fig. 8.15 **a** and **b** TVUS images of diffuse adenomyosis of the anterior wall of the uterus, the uterus is anteverted. (**a**) is a grey-scale ultrasound image showing a marked thickening of the anterior wall of the uterus, significantly uneven echoes, and fan-shaped sound shadows. (**b**) is a color doppler flow imaging (CDFI). The CDFI image shows abundant myometrial blood vessels with increased blood flow signals. (**c** and **d**) TVUS images of focal adenomyosis, the uterine position is also anterior in this case. (**c**) is a grey-scale ultrasound image showing focal lesions with uneven echoes visible in the anterior wall uterine myometrium, and the border is unclear. (**d**) is a CDFI image showing an increase in blood flow signals within the lesion

The CDFI blood flow performance of the two is significantly different. Focal adenomyosis/adenomyoma is a penetrating blood flow mode. In contrast, the typical blood flow pattern of uterine fibroids is a peripheral blood flow mode, which is caused by pressure displacement of blood vessels at the pseudocapsule of the fibroid.

8.4.8 Ultrasound Scanning Skill for Adenomyosis

1. There are complementary imaging effects of the transabdominal probe and transvaginal probe. The transabdominal examination can make a more comprehensive observation of a large uterus. When the uterus is large, high-frequency transvaginal probes can hardly show the uterine muscle layer of the entire posterior wall. At this time, low-frequency transabdominal ultrasound probes should be used. Besides, low-frequency probes can also improve the display of endometrial boundaries.

2. On a single static ultrasound image of adenomyosis, it is sometimes difficult to identify changes in some echogenicities and fan-shaped sound shadows. Using the frame-by-frame playback (cine clips, movie editing) function after the freeze-frame image, these ultrasound features of adenomyosis can be better observed, especially for the uterine JZ layer non-uniformity and fan-shaped sound shadow. Observations are often visible when playing back uterine images frame by frame. It is also easier to observe the continuity of the echo stripes in the endometrial-myometrial JZ through playback.

8.4.9 Ultrasound Uterine Sliding Sign

When using a transvaginal probe, gently push the uterus and ovaries; they slide freely and are positive for sliding signs, indicating that these pelvic organs are non-adhesive; when they are not free to move, they are negative for sliding signs, meaning that the uterus and ovaries have adhesions or may have pelvic endometriosis, etc. [16].

In adenomyosis, if the outer myometrial layer is involved, the serosal layer may be involved as well. In order to determine the involvement of the uterine serosal layer, the uterus should be recorded for slippage or adhesion to the intestine during ultrasound examination; a negative uterine sliding sign indicates adenomyosis may involve the uterine serosa [17].

Of course, the importance of the ultrasound uterine sliding sign lies in the judgment of the entire uterus and pelvic adhesions and whether the adenomyosis is accompanied by deep infiltrating endometriosis at the same time. Because adenomyosis may not be a single manifestation with endometriosis, there may be other endometriosis, such as ovarian endometriosis (chocolate cysts), deep infiltration endometriosis, etc. Ovarian cysts are easier to find by ultrasonography, while deep infiltrating endometriosis may be to ignore during ultrasonography. Careful scanning is required during the examination. In the presence of an ovarian cyst, the application of sliding signs can also detect any adhesion of the cyst to the uterus and surrounding organs.

8.4.10 Ultrasound Classification of Adenomyosis

According to the ultrasound appearances of adenomyosis, they are mainly divided into two types: diffuse adenomyosis and focal adenomyosis.

The ultrasound features of focal adenomyosis can be divided into two subtypes—adenomyoma and cystic adenomyoma. The classification of ultrasound imaging is closely related to the clinical and histopathology of adenomyosis. Histologically, the endometrial glands and interstitial tissue of adenomyosis are diffusely distributed in the muscular layer. When the endometrial glands and interstitials are localized and nodular, with the periphery surrounded by normal myometrium, this lesion is called focal adenomyosis. Both the adenomyoma and cystic adenomyoma are surrounded by a thick layer of the myometrium, with cystic adenomyoma showing cystic changes in the central area of the lesion.

8.4.11 Diffuse Adenomyosis

The posterior uterine wall, uterine fundus, or anterior wall is diffusely involved by adenomyosis. The ultrasound of diffuse adenomyosis is enlarged uterus, and the anterior and posterior walls are often asymmetric. The echogenicity of the affected uterine myometrium is heterogeneous and rough. Fan-shaped sound shadow is common, that is, there are more linear acoustic shadows in the uterine myometrium, and sometimes small cysts (< 5 mm) or microcysts can be seen in the affected myometrium. The boundary between the endometrium and the myometrium is unclear, and high-frequency transvaginal ultrasound sometimes shows moderate-high linear or nodular echo in the JZ zone; CDFI shows increased blood flow signals in the affected myometrium.

8.4.12 Focal Adenomyosis

The focal adenomyosis shows local thickening of the myometrium, heterogeneity, roughness, and fan-shaped sound shadows, sometimes small cysts or microcysts, CDFI seeing blood flow signals in the area of the lesion, and the flow signal can be increased. These ultrasound features of focal adenomyosis are consistent with that of diffuse adenomyosis; there is also an unclear border of the focal lesion (Figure 8.7a, b), and the JZ between the endometrium and the surrounding myometrium is blurred and difficult to distinguish the boundary.

Uterine adenomyoma refers to the focal adenomyosis with relatively clear boundaries. The lesion has a distinguishable border, but it is still not clear enough compared with that of the uterine fibroid (Fig. 8.8).

The cystic adenomyoma is a rare type of focal adenomyosis. It is manifested with old blood-filled cysts in the adenomyoma lesion, and the maximum diameter of the cyst usually exceeds ≥1 cm. Clinical and ultrasound examinations are easily misdiagnosed as residual blood in a uterine horn or cystic changes in a fibroid.

According to the age of onset, the disease can be divided into adolescent and adult types. From the literature [18], it pointed out the diagnostic criteria for adolescent cystic adenomyosis: (1) age ≤ 30 years; (2) the size of the cyst is generally greater than or equal to 1 cm; the cyst cavity is independent of the uterine cavity and the surrounding hyperplastic smooth muscle tissue; and (3) early severe dysmenorrhea. In contrast, the diagnostic criteria for adult type are vague; Kriplani et al. [19] pointed out that the age of onset of adult type is >30 years, the symptoms are similar to typical adenomyosis, and there is a history of uterine surgical trauma.

The size of cystic adenomyoma is mostly 3 to 5 cm in diameter and is located at the posterior wall of the uterus and cornua. Sometimes the lesion is deep and challenging to find with the naked eye, but ultrasound examination may determine the location of the lesion. A cut opened lesion can show chocolate-like fluid flowing out, the wall thickness of the capsule is about 5 to 8 mm, and the diameter of the capsule cavity is mostly 1 to 3 cm, which is not connected with the uterine cavity. The endometrial glands and their interstitium form the cyst wall, which is surrounded by a hypertrophic uterine muscle, forming the cystic adenomyoma.

On the contrary, ultrasound manifestation of cystic adenomyosis showed that it is often located in the uterine myometrium near the cornua of the uterus. There is no clear border, and the uterus is enlarged to varying degrees. There is an anechoic area in the center or hypoechoic area, surrounded by thick hypoechoic areas (Figure 8.16a–d); CDFI can see the sparse star-shaped blood flow signals in the internal solid area [18–20].

Cystic adenomyosis should be distinguished from residual uterine hemorrhage and cystic fibroids. For bleeding in a cornual area, the ultrasound shows that the uterus and uterine cavity are relatively normal, only with a cystic echo in the muscle layer near the uterine cornua. Differentiating it from cystic fibroids can sometimes be difficult. The ultrasound performance of the two is similar and easy to misdiagnose. The main points of identification are a clear boundary of uterine fibroids, and CDFI shows circular blood flow signals around the lesion. In contrast, cystic uterine adenomyoma is unclear, and the peripheral blood flow signal is not apparent.

8.4.13 Differential Diagnosis of Adenomyosis

Uterine adenomyosis needs to be distinguished from uterine fibroid, myometrial contraction, myometrial invasion due to endometrial cancer, and myometrial vascular abnormalities.

8.4.13.1 Uterine Fibroids

Focal adenomyosis and uterine leiomyoma have similar ultrasound performance and need to be identified. It is necessary to distinguish the two accurately. The main

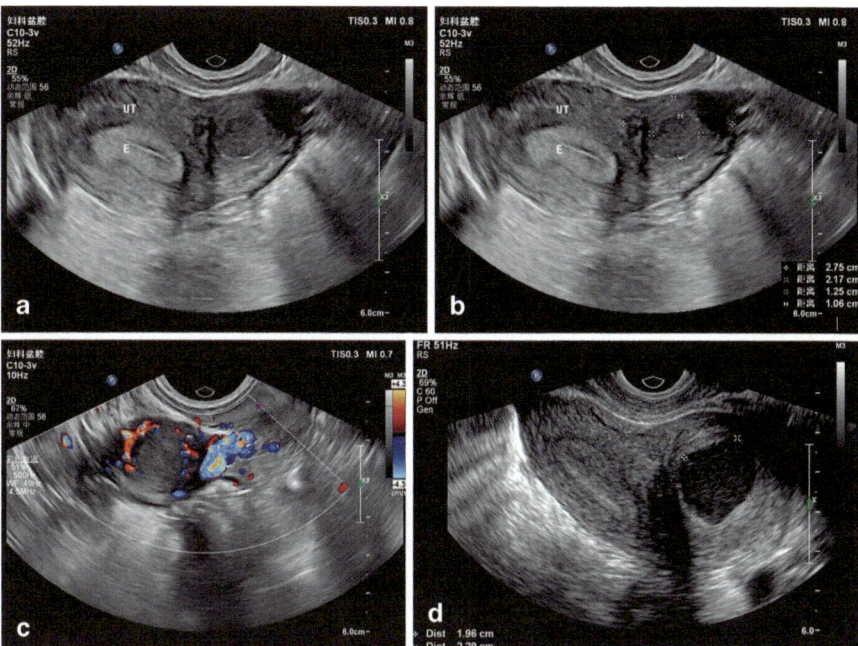

Fig. 8.16 (**a-d**): Transabdominal and transrectal ultrasound images of cystic adenomyosis. (**a-c**) are transabdomianal images with transvaginal probe placed on the abdomen. (**a** and **b**) show a mixed echo mass at the left wall of the uterus near the left corner of the uterus. The central area of the mass is a non-echo area with poor sound transmission. Thick echogenic areas are surrounding the anechoic area. In the hypoechoic area, the size of the entire lesion is 2.8 cm × 2.2 cm, and the size of the non-echo area is 1.3 cm × 1.1 cm. The boundary between the lesion and the normal muscular layer is unclear. (**c**) is a CDFI image of this case, showing a surrounding blood flow signal around the lesion. (**d**) is a transrectal ultrasound image of this case at the time of re-examination 10 months later. It can be seen that the frost glass in the non-echoic area of the center of the lesion is more typical, with a size of 2.3 cm × 2.0 cm

points of adenomyosis and uterine leiomyoma are their borders, features of small cysts, and internal echoes as well as the appearance of CDFI. Uterine fibroids have pseudocapsules, which appear as well-defined masses, sometimes in concentric circles or swirls. The echogenicities of uterine fibroids vary widely, from uniform hypoechoic, iso-echogenic, or high echogenic to unevenly mixed echoes and/or hyperechoic (calcification), etc.; the blood flow of fibroids is mainly peripheral (Figure 8.17a, b).

In contrast, the border of uterine adenomyoma is unclear, and it is mostly hypoechoic. The blood flow is dominantly penetrating blood flow (Figure 8.18a, b). CDFI plays a crucial role in distinguishing uterine fibroids from adenomyomas. Chiang et al. 1999 [15] reported that 88% of adenomyosis is penetrating blood flow, and 87% of leiomyomas are peripheral blood flow. When identification is difficult, contrast-enhanced ultrasound can help define the diagnosis. Also, leiomyoma and adenomyosis both have a fan-shaped sound shadow. However, the sound shadow of uterine fibroids tends to be uneven and irregular, and the sound shadow of

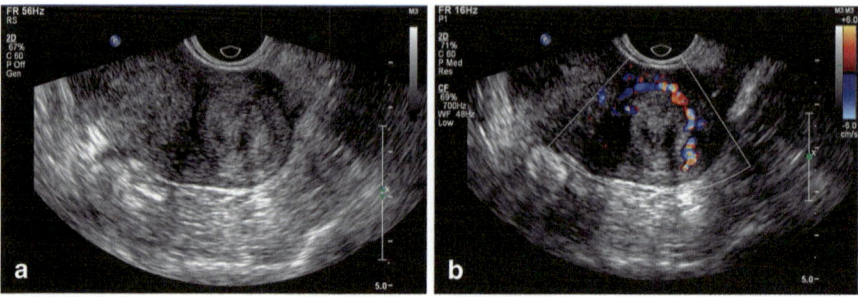

Fig. 8.17 (**a** and **b**) TVUS images of uterine fibroids, the uterus is retroverted. (**a**) is a grey-scale ultrasound image showing the hypoechoic lesion visible at the fundus of the uterus, with regular morphology and clear boundaries; (**b**) is a CDFI image showing a typical circular blood flow signal around the uterine lesion

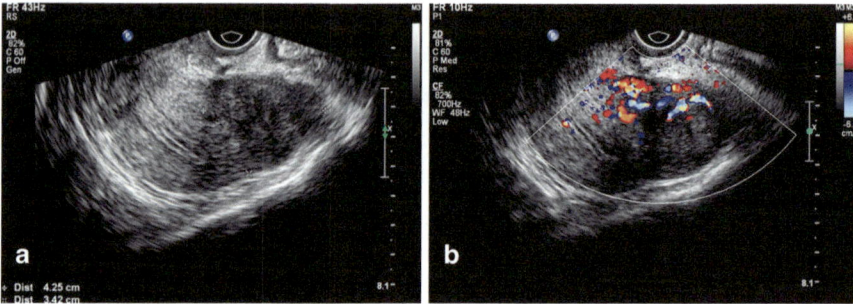

Fig. 8.18 (**a** and **b**): TVUS images of focal adenomyosis in the posterior wall of the uterus, the uterus is retroverted. (**a**) is a grey-scale ultrasound image showing a hypoechoic area seen in the posterior wall of the uterus, protruding towards the surface of the uterus, with unclear boundaries, and the echo in the lesion is significantly uneven. (**b**) is a CDFI image showing a typical penetrating blood flow signal into the uterine lesion

adenomyosis tend to be even and fine. It should be noted that uterine fibroids and adenomyosis are common diseases and often coexist.

8.4.13.2 Myometrial Contraction

The contraction of the myometrium can sometimes be expressed as a focal hypoechoic mass in the myometrium, which can be mistaken for uterine fibroids or focal adenomyosis, requiring the attention of young physicians to make a diagnosis. The local contraction of the myometrium can be distinguished from the myometrial lesion by its short-term nature, and it can be identified by re-examination by ultrasound in about half an hour later.

8.4.13.3 Myometrial Infiltration of Endometrial Cancer

Endometrial cancer may also be irregular when the myometrium invades the muscular layer and needs to be identified. Endometrial cancer is characterized by endometrial thickening and abundant local blood flow. When invading the myometrium, the uterine JZ under the endometrium is destroyed, like adenomyosis. CDFI shows the local increase in endometrial blood flow. According to the thickening of the endometrium, the affected JZ and the muscle layer have a more clumpy effect, unlike the thin stripes and small island nodules of adenomyosis. MRI evaluation and endometrial biopsy can confirm the diagnosis [21].

8.5 Application of New Ultrasound Technology in the Diagnosis and Treatment of Adenomyosis

8.5.1 Application of 3D Ultrasound

The most important value of 3D ultrasound in diagnosing adenomyosis is that it can more intuitively show the endometrial-muscular JZ, which can diagnose adenomyosis early, because the uterine JZ is the earliest ectopic endometrial lesion. The appearance shows either an enlarged or discontinued JZ observed by the 3D ultrasound scan. The application of 3D ultrasound post-processing technology (VCI technology) can improve the contrast of the image and better display the JZ [22].

3D ultrasound features of adenomyosis also include irregular bands, thickening, interruptions, sub-endometrial hyperechoic lines, and island nodules in the JZ similar to the 2D ultrasound features [3, 11, 14, 22].

8.5.2 Application of Elastography

Elastography has been used in the diagnosis of many organs and systems. The literature shows that the sensitivity and specificity of elastography in diagnosing adenomyosis is 89.7% and 92.9%. The stiffness and hardness of the adenomyosis are much higher than that of a normal myometrium, which is closely related to the fibrosis of the adenomyosis tissues. The lesional stiffness detected by elastography in the adenomyosis correlated with hormone receptor expression levels, which is also related to the severity of pain symptoms [23, 24]. However, Zhang et al. 2019 [25] showed that elastography did not distinguish between fibroids and adenomyosis. It can be seen that the application of elastography in adenomyosis requires further research, and it is still difficult to use it for routine diagnosis [25].

New Advances in the Diagnosis of Adenomyosis by Ultrasound.

More and more research evidence show that adenomyosis is closely related to infertility. Although the mechanism is unknown, early diagnosis and evaluation can help to preserve female reproductive function. The more extensive ultrasound features of adenomyosis, the more likely it indicates a higher risk of infertility. Some scholars have proposed a scoring system to assess the severity of adenomyosis, which specifically corresponds to the severity of ultrasound signs and guides for individualized treatment [26].

Many studies have pointed out the need to clarify the role of changes in the uterine JZ in the diagnosis of adenomyosis and emphasized the need to obtain good images of the zone through 3D transvaginal ultrasound [3, 11, 14, 22]. 3D ultrasound may also need to be involved in clinical practice to make an early diagnosis of adenomyosis and hopefully to treat the adenomyosis and conserve fertility in its early development.

Ultrasound diagnosis for adenomyosis depends to some extent on the experience of the examiner. In recent years, some scholars have proposed the need for standardized training of ultrasound residents and to improve the diagnosis of adenomyosis through standardized pattern recognition learning. They have also suggested the use of ultrasound feature checklists to promote pattern recognition learning [22, 27].

European and American ultrasound scholars discussed it in a meeting and reached a consensus recommendation. They proposed a standardized and unified classification and reporting system for adenomyosis [28]. The consensus recommends that ultrasound reports for adenomyosis should include seven points:

1. According to the 2015 publication of the Uterine Ultrasound Evaluation Research Group (MUSA), the consensus of MUSA established the standardized terms, definitions, and measurements of the ultrasound characteristics of the uterine myometrium and uterine mass, to set up the criteria for identifying adenomyosis [29].
2. The location of the lesion (anterior wall, posterior wall, left side wall, right side wall, outer sidewall, and uterine fundus).
3. Focal or diffuse lesions: more than 25% of myometrial involvement of the uterine body is classified as diffuse adenomyosis; if it is difficult to distinguish between focal and diffuse lesions, the lesion should be reported as diffuse adenomyosis; if there are both diffuse and focal adenomyosis in different parts of the uterus, it is called "hybrid adenomyosis." Focal adenomyosis is defined as an adenomyoma of the uterus when it is surrounded by a thick layer of the myometrium, with relatively clear boundaries.
4. The definition of cystic adenomyoma is the presence of measurable cysts inside the adenomyosis. Generally, the maximum diameter is at least 2 mm, which is always measurable. It should be reported if the cysts are present in all types of adenomyosis (focal, diffuse, mixed adenomyosis, and adenomyoma).
5. Assessing the involvement of various layers of the uterus, including the uterine JZ, the uterine muscle layer, and the serosa layer.
6. Degree of the disease (adenomyosis affects uterine volume < 25%, 25–50%, >50%): subjective assessment of disease severity (mild <25%, moderate 25–50%, or severe >50% adenomyosis).
7. The size of the lesion: for diffuse lesions, there is a need to measure the thickness of the anterior and posterior wall of the uterus. For focal lesions, at least the maximum diameter of each lesion should be measured. The three diameters of the lesion should be recorded when conducting research.

The consensus statement [28] issued by MUSA in 2015 suggested that standardized terms should be used to describe ultrasound images of adenomyosis. However, it did not guide the classification or degree of adenomyosis. UOG in 2018 issued this classification, and the reporting system [29] helps to compensate for the deficiency, which is worth our attention. Of course, the clinical application of this classification and reporting system needs further confirmation and improvement.

To summarize, ultrasound is the clinically preferred imaging method for adenomyosis, and transvaginal ultrasound is the main ultrasound examination for diagnosing adenomyosis. In most cases, transvaginal ultrasound can more accurately diagnose adenomyosis, especially when there are multiple ultrasound features of adenomyosis; ultrasound has higher effectiveness in diagnosing adenomyosis. The 2D ultrasound playback function and advanced ultrasound technology, such as the reconstructed image of 3D ultrasound, can supplement the deficiency of conventional ultrasound and further improve the diagnostic efficacy of ultrasound for adenomyosis.

References

1. Bohlman ME, Ensor RE, Sanders RC. Sonographic findings in adenomyosis of the uterus. AJR Am J Roentgenol. 1987;148(4):765–6.
2. Tan J, Yong P, Bedaiwy MA. A critical review of recent advances in the diagnosis, classification, and management of uterine adenomyosis. Curr Opin Obstet Gynecol. 2019;31:212–21.
3. Rasmussen CK, Hansen ES, Dueholm M. Two- and three-dimensional ultrasonographic features related to histopathology of the uterine endometrial-myometrial junctional zone. Acta Obstet Gynecol Scand. 2019;98(2):205–14.
4. Karamanidis D, Nicolaou P, Chrysafis I, et al. Transvaginal ultrasonography compared with magnetic resonance imaging for the diagnosis of adenomyosis. Ultrasound Obstet Gynecol. 2018;52(4):555–6.
5. Champaneria R, Abedin P, Daniels J, Balogun M, Khan KS. Ultrasound scan and magnetic resonance imaging for the diagnosis of adenomyosis: systematic review comparing test accuracy. Acta Obstet Gynecol Scand. 2010;89:1374–84.
6. Van den Bosch T, Van Schoubroeck D. Ultrasound diagnosis of endometriosis and adenomyosis: state of the art. Best Pract Res Clin Obstet Gynaecol. 2018;51:16–24.
7. Cunningham RK, Horrow MM, Smith RJ, et al. Adenomyosis: A Sonographic diagnosis. Radio Graphics. 2018;38(5):576–1589.
8. Konrad J, Merck D, Wu JY, et al. Improving ultrasound detection of uterine Adenomyosis through computational texture analysis. Ultrasound Q. 2017;34(1):29–31.
9. Tellum T, Nygaard S, Skovholt EK, et al. Development of a clinical prediction model for diagnosing adenomyosis. Fertil Steril. 2018;110(5):957–64. e3
10. Pinzauti S, Lazzeri L, Tostic C, et al. Transvaginal sonographic features of diffuse adenomyosis in 18–30-year-old nulligravid women without endometriosis: association with symptoms. Ultrasound Obstet Gynecol. 2015;46:730–6.
11. Votino A. Van den Bosc h T, Installé AJF et al. optimizing the ultrasound visualization of the endometrial-myometrial junction (EMJ). Facts Views Vis Obgyn. 2015;7(1):60–3.
12. Kepkep K, Tuncay YA, Goynumer G, Tutal E. Transvaginal sonography in the diagnosis of adenomyosis: which findings are most accurate? Ultrasound Obstet Gynecol. 2007;30:341–5.
13. Bazot M, Cortez A, Darai E, et al. Ultrasonography compared with magnetic resonance imaging for the diagnosis of adenomyosis: correlation with histopathology. Hum Reprod. 2001;16(11):2427–33.

14. Exacoustos C, Brienza L, Di Giovanni A, et al. Adenomyosis: three-dimensional sonographic findings of the junctional zone and correlation with histology. Ultrasound Obstet Gynecol. 2011;37:471–9.
15. Chiang CH, Chang MY, Hsu JJ, et al. Tumor vascular pattern and blood flow impedance in the differential diagnosis of leiomyoma and adenomyosis by color Doppler sonography. J Assist Reprod Genet. 1999;16(5):268–75.
16. Reid S, Condous G. Transvaginal sonographic sliding sign: accurate prediction of pouch f Douglas obliteration. Ultrasound Obstet Gynecol. 2013;41:605–7.
17. Groszmann YS, Benacerraf BR. Complete evaluation of anatomy and morphology of the infertile patient in a single visit; the modern infertility pelvic ultrasound examination. Fertil Steril. 2016;105:1381–93.
18. Takeuchi H, Kitade M, Kikuchi I, et al. Diagnosis, laparoscopic management, and histopathologic findings of juvenile cystic adenomyoma: a review of nine cases. Fertil Steril. 2010;94:862–8.
19. Kriplani A, Mahey R, Agarwal N, et al. Laparoscopic management of juvenile cystic adenomyoma: four cases. J Minim Invasive Gynecol. 2011;18:343–8.
20. Nabeshima H, Murakami T, Nishimoto M, et al. Successful total laparoscopic cystic adenomyomectomy after unsuccessful open surgery using transtrocar ultrasonographic guiding. J Minim Invasive Gynecol. 2008;15:227–30.
21. Puente JM, Fabris A, Patel J, et al. Adenomyosis in infertile women prevalence and the role of 3D ultrasound as a marker of severity of the disease. Reprod Biol Endocrinol. 2016;14:60.
22. Rasmussen CK, Hansen ES, Dueholm M. Inter-rater agreement in the diagnosis of Adenomyosis by 2 and 3-dimensional Transvaginal ultrasonography. J Ultrasound Med. 2019;38:657–65.
23. Liu X, Ding D, Ren Y, et al. Transvaginal Elastosonography as an imaging technique for diagnosing Adenomyosis. Reprod Sci. 2018;25(4):498–514.
24. Acar S, Millar E, Mitkova M, et al. Value of ultrasound shear wave elastography in the diagnosis of adenomyosis. Ultrasound. 2016;24(4):205–13.
25. Zhang M, Wasnik AP, Masch WR, et al. Transvaginal ultrasound shear wave Elastography for the evaluation of benign uterine pathologies: A prospective pilot study. J Ultrasound Med. 2019;38(1):149–55.
26. Lazzeri L, Morosetti G, Centini G, et al. A sonographic classification of adenomyosis: interobserver reproducibility in the evaluation of type and degree of the myometrial involvement. Fertil Steril. 2018;110(6):1154–1161.e3.
27. Eisenberg, VH, Arbib N, Schiff E, et al. Sonographic Signs of Adenomyosis Are Prevalent in Women Undergoing Surgery for Endometriosis and May Suggest a Higher Risk of Infertility. BioMed Research International, 2017. http://doi.org/10.1155/2017/8967803.
28. Van den Bosch T, de BRUIJN AM, A de LEEUW R, et al. A sonographic classification and reporting system for diagnosing adenomyosis. Ultrasound Obst Gyn. 2018;22(5):764.
29. Van den Bosch T, Dueholm M, Leone FP, et al. Terms, definitions and measurements to describe sonographic features of myometrium and uterine masses: a consensus opinion from the morphological uterus Sonographic assessment (MUSA)group. Ultrasound Obstet Gynecol. 2015;46(3):284–98.

Magnetic Resonance Imaging Manifestations and Classification of Adenomyosis

9

Jingjing Lu and Jinhua Leng

Magnetic resonance imaging (MRI) is one of the important imaging methods for the female reproductive system. In recent years, its application in the management of adenomyosis has been increasingly recognized by clinical physicians. MRI has been mainly applied to the diagnosis, typing, and monitoring after treatment of uterine adenomyosis due to its many advantages, such as clear and intuitive images, operator-independent features, and multi-parameter and multi-planar techniques. Since imaging diagnosis is now essential for a comprehensive diagnosis of adenomyosis, MRI has been increasingly applied to make a diagnosis, typing, and monitoring the treatment result of adenomyosis. The gradual popularization of MRI equipment, the decline in scanning costs, and the rapid development of its software and hardware have also increased its application. This chapter mainly describes the basic MRI manifestations, classification, and findings of each subtype of adenomyosis and introduces the relevant MRI technology and application frontiers.

9.1 The Basic MRI Manifestations and Classification of Adenomyosis

The classic appearance of MRI for adenomyosis is the diffuse enlargement of the uterus, generally with smooth outer contours, with the lesions more clearly displayed on the T2-weighted image. They are low-signal lesions with poorly defined borders, adjacent to the endometrium, and unclear boundaries. Sometimes it may

J. Lu (✉)
Department of Radiology/Imaging, Beijing United Family Hospital, Beijing, China
e-mail: cjr.lujingjing@vip.163.com

J. Leng
Department of Obstetrics and Gynecology, Peking Union Medical College Hospital, Beijing, China

manifest as a thickening or distortion of the endometrial–myometrial junctional zone (JZ); multiple spot-like hyperintense signals are often seen in the lesion, and these spot-like signals correspond histopathologically to the hyperplasia of endometrial tissue in the ectopic foci, with or without accompanying changes of the bleeding. The surrounding low-signal areas correspond to the proliferation of the smooth muscle and fibrous tissue. MRI T2-weighted image of adenomyosis (Fig. 9.1) shows slightly blurred lesion with no sharp boundary, but focal tissues with bleeding can show hyperintense cystic signals [1].

Adenomyosis has a variety of presentations due to its involvement in different parts of the uterus and its histopathological basis [1–3]. Therefore, scholars have also tried to type the magnetic resonance manifestations of adenomyosis to facilitate systematic interpretation and communication. Kishi et al. proposed in 2012 to divide adenomyosis into four subtypes according to the MRI appearances [4]: Subtype I is called internal (intrinsic) adenomyosis, which means that adenomyosis occurs only in the inner layer of the uterus. The lesion shows a thickened endometrium–myometrial JZ but does not involve the outer uterine layer. Subtype II is called external (extrinsic) adenomyosis, which occurs only in the outer layer of the uterus and does not involve the JZ. Subtype III is called adenomyoma (intramural), which exists alone in the myometrial layer and does not involve other structures (Fig. 9.2). Subtype IV includes adenomyosis that cannot be identified as any of the above three subtypes, and it has a mixed presentation.

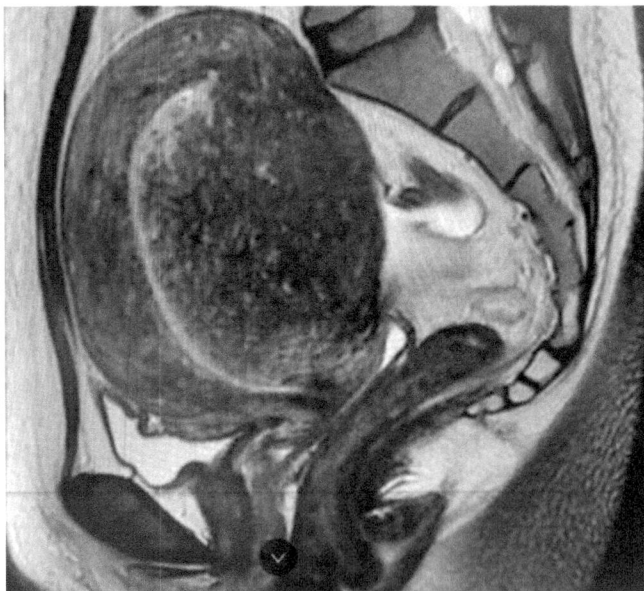

Fig. 9.1 MRI T2W image of posterior adenomyosis showing no sharp boundary, with hyperintense cystic signals in the lesion

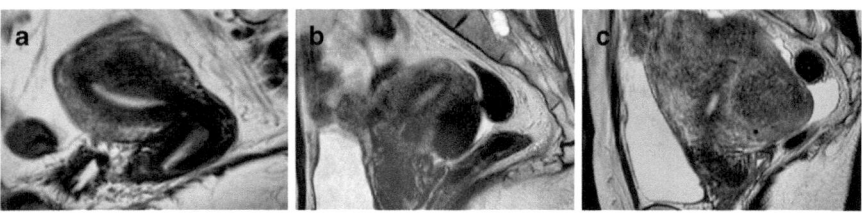

Fig. 9.2 Subtypes I-III of adenomyosis in MRI images. (**a**) Internal (intrinsic) adenomyosis, (**b**) External (extrinsic) adenomyosis, (**c**) Adenomyoma (intramural)

Table 9.1 Types of adenomyosis (reproduced with permission from [3])

Definition of adenomyosis subtype	Definition	Figure
Internal adenomyosis(Ai)		
Focal adenomyosis(Ai0)	Localized intramyometrial cystic component with or without JZ bulging (unique or multiple)	1A
Superficial adenomyosis (Ai1)	Disseminated subendometrial tiny cystic component without JZ hypertrophy (symmetric or asymmetric)	1B, 1C
Diffuse adenomyosis (Ai2)	Disseminated intramyometrial tiny cystic component with JZ hypertrophy (symmetric or asymmetric)	1D, 1E
Adenomyoma(ad)		
Intramural solid adenomyoma (Ad1)	An ill-defined myometrial lesion with tiny cystic component (hemorrhagic or not)	1F
Intramural cystic adenomyoma (Ad2)	An ill-defined myometrial lesion with hemorrhagic cystic activities	1G
Submucosal adenomyoma (Ad3)	An ill-defined myometrial lesion with tiny cystic component and intracavity protrusion	1H
Subserosal adenomyoma (Ad4)	An ill-defined subserosal myometrial lesion with tiny cystic components	1I
External adenomyosis (Ae)		
Posterior external adenomyosis (Ae1)	An ill-defined subserosal posterior myometrial mass associated with posterior deep endometriosis	1 J
Anterior external adenomyosis (Ae2)	An ill-defined subserosal anterior myometrial mass associated with anterior deep endometriosis	1 K

The significance of this subtype classification is to suggest the different pathogenesis of adenomyosis. Subtype I represents the direct invasion of the endometrium, subtype II represents the invasion of the ectopic endometrium from the outside, subtype III represents the in-situ endometrial metaplasia, and subtype IV is the sum of a group of more progressive disease forms.

Bazot et al. 2018 [3] defined the MRI classification of adenomyosis based on predecessors' classification into three types: internal adenomyosis, external adenomyosis, and anatomical-related adenomyoma. It is according to different forms of adenomyosis, uterine location, and possible treatment criteria, and they further subdivide the entity into 11 subtypes, from A to K [3]. This classification is relatively complicated, and though it is the latest and comprehensive classification (Table 9.1, Fig. 9.3 and 9.4), its acceptance still needs more clinical appraisal in the future.

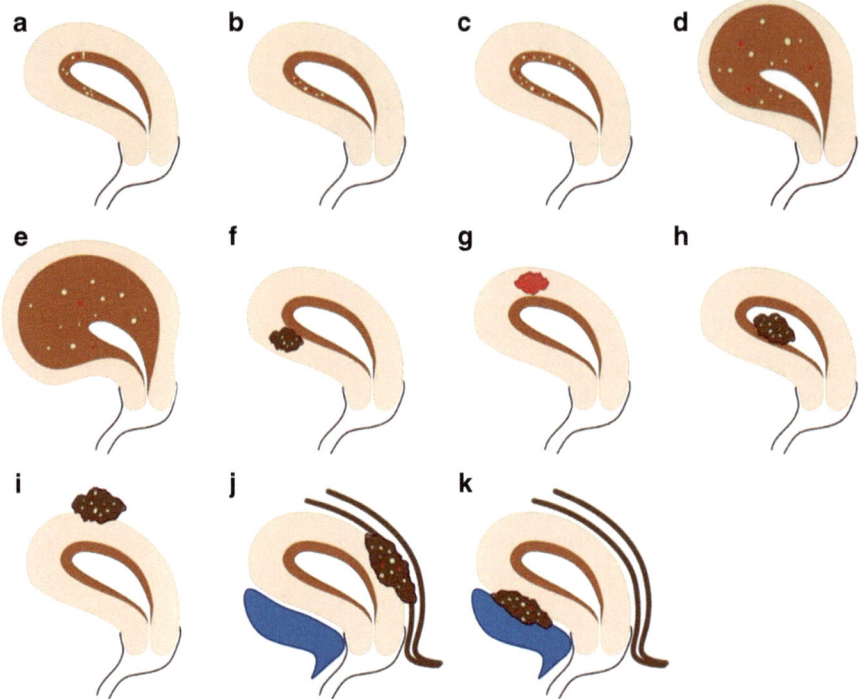

Fig. 9.3 MRI classification of adenomyosis, which is typed by Bazot et al. according to the different morphology and location of the adenomyosis, including internal adenomyosis, adenomyoma, and external adenomyosis. There are 11 subtypes from A to K, which correspond to the subtype descriptions in Table 9.1 (Fig. 9.3 is reproduced with permission from reference [3])

9.2 MRI Appearances of Different Subtypes of Adenomyosis

9.2.1 Internal Adenomyosis

Internal adenomyosis refers to ectopic endometrial hyperplasia under the endometrium or superficial myometrium, with the tiny cystic changes, and the surrounding smooth muscle hypertrophy in the adenomyosis. The main MRI signs are multiple small intramuscular cysts with smooth muscle hyperplasia and ill-defined surrounding boundaries (Fig. 9.2a to e). Multiple small cystic lesions are generally less than 3 mm in diameter (Fig. 9.2a). These cystic lesions are embedded in the muscular layer, mainly the inner muscular layer, with high signals on the T2-weighted image and low signals on the T1-weighted image [1]. This sign is a direct, specific sign of adenomyosis but only in about 50% of patients [5].

Indirect signs of internal adenomyosis are focal or diffuse thickening of the JZ, which occur more often than direct signs. MRI can clearly show the JZ, so it plays a very important role in the diagnosis of internal adenomyosis. The JZ is defined as a continuous low-signal zone between the high-signal endometrium and the

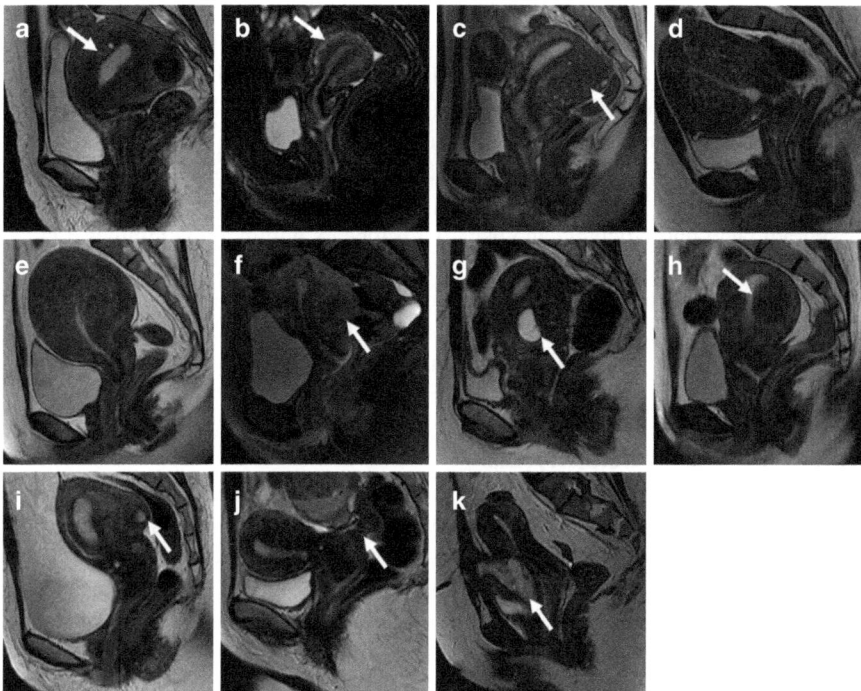

Fig. 9.4 MRI manifestations of various types of adenomyosis (corresponding to the various types in Fig. 9.1): A to E are internal adenomyosis, F to I are adenomyoma, and J to K are external adenomyosis (reproduced with permission reference)

medium-signal outer muscle layer on the T2-weighted image of MRI. It is confirmed by pathology to correspond with the innermost layer of the muscle layer, without the basal layer of the intima [6]. The JZ presents in the T1-weighted image as a slightly higher signal zone between the low-signal intima and the middle-signal outer muscle layer, which is most clearly shown on the fat-saturated T1-weighted image [3]. Histologically, the endometrium and the JZ are derived from the Mullerian duct, while the outer muscle layer is derived from non-Mullerian-derived stroma [7].

The width of the normal JZ was considered to be the widest thickness between 5 mm and 8 mm in early studies, and the most important MRI criterion for diagnosing adenomyosis is that the thickness of the JZ is greater than or equal to 12 mm (Fig. 9.2a, d, e). Several studies have found that the sensitivity of this criterion to diagnose adenomyosis is 63%–93%, and the specificity is 88%–96% [3].

The morphological features of the JZ are also affected by many factors, such as physiology and drug treatment. Pseudo thickening of the JZ can often be found during menstruation, and it can be found during the pre-menstrual period, pregnancy, menopause, and treatment with GnRH-a; there may be a poor display of JZ. For females undergoing hormone replacement therapy after menopause, JZ can reappear. According to statistics, 20%–30% of women of childbearing age and more than 50% of postmenopausal women show unclear JZs. Therefore, in the diagnosis of adenomyosis with MRI evaluation of JZs, it is necessary to consider the various phases of the menstrual cycle, physiology, and medication [7]. Besides, the presence of fibroids often affects the observation of the JZ. The JZ plays a major role in the peristalsis of the uterus. Normal uterine peristalsis is a continuous and periodic phenomenon that is distinguished from uterine contraction. The uterine contraction is sporadic and unpredictable and usually disappears within a few minutes. On the T2-weighted image, it can appear as isolated or multiple, focal, or diffuse low-signal areas. Frequently, uterine contraction needs to be differentiated from internal adenomyosis, adenomyoma, and fibroids. Fast T2-weighted sequences can often track the disappearance of this contraction over time [3, 8].

9.2.2 External Adenomyosis

This subtype occurs mainly in the posterior part of the uterus (96.1%) and is often accompanied by teardrop-like deformation of the rectum. Besides, it is often associated with endometriosis, which can be found in most patients during surgery, with pouch of Douglas (POD) closure (96.1%), pelvic endometriosis (92.2%), and ovarian chocolate cysts (66.7%) [3]. This finding strongly suggests that this subtype is homologous to pelvic endometriosis in its pathogenesis [9].

Local fibrous tissue hyperplasia due to POD endometriosis leads to adhesion of surrounding structures, partial or complete closure of the POD, thickening of the uterosacral ligaments, and invasion of the rectum, causing teardrop-like traction and deformation, and forward involvement of the uterine serosa (Fig. 9.2j) leads to external adenomyoma which forms a classic "hourglass"-like appearance.

The MRI manifestations of this subtype lesion are low or low to moderate signal masses with poorly defined borders (small spot-like high signals caused by bleeding are often seen inside), which are asymmetrically located in the outer muscular layer of the posterior uterus, making the posterior wall of the uterus bulging. At the same time, the JZ is intact, and the muscle layer tissue between the lesion and the JZ remains as normal [4]. Relatively rarely, this subtype is a lesion involving the anterior pelvis, that is, a deep adenomyoma located in the space between the anterior muscular layer and the bladder (Fig. 9.2k).

9.2.3 Adenomyoma

Adenomyoma appears on the T2-weighted image as a low-signaled lesion in the muscle layer with an ill-defined border and may contain small cystic foci with high signals. Sometimes small cystic foci appear brighter on the T1-weighted image [10]. Neither the JZ nor the uterine serosa was involved by adenomyoma [4]. MRI can accurately show the anatomical location of adenomyoma (intermuscular (Fig. 9.2f, g), submucosal (Fig. 9.2h), or subserosal (Fig. 9.2i)), the number and its relationship with internal adenomyosis or leiomyoma, as well as its potential connection with these tumors.

In the diagnosis of adenomyoma with MRI, care must be taken to distinguish between leiomyoma and myometrial contraction. Persistent uterine muscle contraction is manifested by local or diffuse bulging of the myometrium in the uterine cavity. Continuous dynamic acquisition of MRI can find its existence temporarily, to distinguish it from adenomyoma or fibroids [2].

Adenomyoma can also be cystic (Fig. 9.2g), with internal hemorrhagic contents. On the T1-weighted image, it is usually a uniform high signal, and on the T2-weighted image, different signals are displayed with varying phases of the menstrual bleeding cycle. Sometimes liquid–liquid planes and low signal edges can be seen on T2-weighted images [11]. This manifestation of adenomyoma must often be distinguished from fibroid degeneration, which is recognized by the fact that the latter tends to have more inhomogeneous signals. Besides, when there is periodic bleeding of the ectopic endometrium and it is not connected with the uterine cavity, a hemorrhagic cystic lesion in the muscular layer can be formed. Other deformity-related morphological changes may occur and be identified.

9.3   The Progressive Development of MRI Technology that Might Be Related to Study Adenomyosis

9.3.1   Cinema Magnetic Resonance Imaging (Cine-MRI)

Conventional MRI technology mainly displays the static morphology of the uterus, which has low time resolution and long image acquisition time and is not suitable for observing weak endometrial peristalsis and muscle layer contraction. On conventional T2-weighted images, focal uterine contractions may be mistaken for uterine fibroids or adenomyoma, resulting in overdiagnosis and treatment. Cine-MRI can acquire MR image using a quick scan sequence, which clearly shows the fine endometrial peristalsis and the spread of peristaltic waves to the outer muscular layer, as well as the changes in uterine morphology and function caused by the contraction of the uterine muscular layer. It will identify a variety of diseases, such as local uterine contractions, adenomyosis, fibroids, and endometriosis [12]. The cine-MRI technology can dynamically observe the contraction and peristalsis of the uterus under physiological and pathological conditions. Therefore it may provide a possible explanation for the pathogenesis of a variety of diseases, such as the abnormal endometrial peristalsis, uterine fibroids, and intrauterine adhesions, postpartum uterine involution with peristalsis, and dysmenorrhea with abnormal peristalsis [13]. The uterine peristaltic movements are generally used for cine-MRI research study.

9.3.2   Diffusion-Weighted Imaging (DWI)

DWI can detect Brownian motion of water molecules in the human body. The diffusion motion of free water is random. Because of the membrane, dense tissue cells, and macromolecules, will interfere with the random motion of water molecules in the body, thereby limiting its Brownian motion. Conventional MRI equipment uses gradients (b-values) of different amplitudes to separate the diffusion characteristics of the tissue to distinguish between diseased tissue and normal tissue. The limit of the diffusion of water molecules in biological tissues is inversely related to the degree of tissue-rich cells and the integrity of cell membranes. Several studies have used DWI to find significant differences in the apparent diffusion coefficients of adenomyosis, fibroids, and the myometrium, which means that in cases where conventional MRI is difficult to distinguish, DWI can provide more evidence for differential diagnosis of these tumors [2].

9.3.3 T2 Mapping

Quantitative magnetic resonance techniques, such as T2 mapping can also be used to study adenomyosis. T2 mapping technology is a magnetic resonance quantitative technique for measuring the T2 value of tissues. In a magnetic resonance scan, a multi-echo spin-echo sequence or a multi-echo fast spin-echo sequence is used to obtain more than two contrast images, and the T2 value can be calculated through calculation. T2 mapping technology can be used in various systems throughout the body, mainly in the bone and joint system, heart, and liver. Recently, researchers have applied this technology to show the layered structure of the uterus and found that T2 mapping technology can use T2 time to show the four layers of the uterus, and found that the outer muscular layer of patients with adenomyosis is thickened as a new imaging sign of adenomyosis [14]. The application is still in the early exploration stage, and the future value needs to be further explored.

9.3.4 MRI Diffusion Tensor Imaging (DTI)

DTI is a new technology that uses diffusion-weighted imaging technology to improve and develop imaging. The diffusion tensor is not a planar process. However, it is decomposed in a three-dimensional angle, which quantifies the signal data of the diffusion anisotropy and makes the microstructure of the tissue more finely displayed. Diffusion needs to be displayed using tensors, and multiple gradient field directions are applied when scanning, often reaching 10 to dozens of directions. This technique is most commonly used in the delineation of neurological diseases and white matter fiber bundles. It is now gradually being applied to the pelvic cavity, mainly the sacral plexus nerve [15]. Some researchers used DTI to scan the sacral plexus nerve roots of women with endometriosis or adenomyosis and analyzed the correlation between the abnormal parameters and pain displayed by DTI and the lesions found during the operation. DTI showed abnormalities of the sacral plexus nerve root microstructure, irregular nerve fibers, and unidirectional walking damage in 66.7% of patients; these abnormalities were found to be associated with dysmenorrhea, acyclic pelvic pain, pain duration, pelvic adhesions, and deep endometriosis. There were significant correlations [16]. This study suggests that DTI may play an important role in the diagnosis and treatment planning of pain caused by endometriosis or adenomyosis.

In summary, with the accumulation of application experience using MRI, the advancement of equipment and technology, MRI will play an increasingly important role in the diagnosis of adenomyosis, monitoring of treatment effects, preoperative planning, and postoperative follow-up.

References

1. Togashi K, et al. Adenomyosis: diagnosis with MR imaging. Radiology. 1988;166(1):111–4.
2. Tamai K, et al. MR imaging findings of adenomyosis: correlation with histopathologic features and diagnostic pitfalls. Radiographics. 2005;25(1):21–40.
3. Bazot M, Daraï E. Role of transvaginal sonography and magnetic resonance imaging in the diagnosis of uterine adenomyosis. Fertil Steril. 2018;109(3):389–97.
4. Kishi Y, et al. Four subtypes of adenomyosis assessed by magnetic resonance imaging and their specification. Am J Obstet Gynecol. 2012;207(2):114–e1-114. e7.
5. Bazot M, et al. Ultrasonography compared with magnetic resonance imaging for the diagnosis of adenomyosis: correlation with histopathology. Hum Reprod. 2001;16(11):2427–33.
6. Novellas S, et al. MRI characteristics of the uterine junctional zone: from normal to the diagnosis of adenomyosis. Am J Roentgenol. 2011;196(5):1206–13.
7. Brosens JJ, de Souza NM, Barker FG. Uterine junctional zone: function and disease. Lancet. 1995;346(8974):558–60.
8. Bazot M, et al. Fast breath-hold T2-weighted MR imaging reduces interobserver variability in the diagnosis of adenomyosis. Am J Roentgenol. 2003;180(5):1291–6.
9. Chapron C, et al. Relationship between the magnetic resonance imaging appearance of adenomyosis and endometriosis phenotypes. Hum Reprod. 2017;32(7):1393–401.
10. Song SE, et al. MR imaging features of uterine adenomyomas. Abdom Imaging. 2011;36(4):483–8.
11. Troiano RN, Flynn SD, McCarthy S. Cystic adenomyosis of the uterus: MRI. J Magn Reson Imaging. 1998;8(6):1198–202.
12. Kido A, Togashi K. Uterine anatomy and function on cine magnetic resonance imaging. Reproductive medicine and biology. 2016;15(4):191–9.
13. Qu Yalin LF, Zhibo X, Fajin L, Hui X, Jia L, Feifei Z. Cine MRI study of uterine peristalsis in patients with fibroids and menorrhagia. Magn Reson Imaging. 2016;7(7):506–11.
14. Ghosh A, et al. T2 relaxometry mapping in demonstrating layered uterine architecture: parameter optimization and utility in endometrial carcinoma and adenomyosis: a feasibility study. Br J Radiol. 2018;91(1081):20170377.
15. Manganaro L, et al. Diffusion tensor imaging and tractography to evaluate sacral nerve root abnormalities in endometriosis-related pain: a pilot study. Eur Radiol. 2014;24(1):95–101.
16. Porpora MG, et al. The role of magnetic resonance imaging–diffusion tensor imaging in predicting pain related to endometriosis: a preliminary study. J Minim Invasive Gynecol. 2018;25(4):661–9.

The Medical Treatment of Adenomyosis

10

Jinghua Shi, Yi Dai, and Jinhua Leng

Uterine adenomyosis is a chronic disease that affects women of childbearing age from years to decades. Conservative surgeries are difficult to perform, and the lesions are prone to recurrence after surgery. They require long-term management. As one of the important issues of long-term management, drug therapy is useful and has effects on controlling symptoms, delaying the progress of the disease, and preventing recurrence. According to the different mechanisms of action, the indications for medication should be understood, used alone or in combination with surgical treatment and integrated traditional Chinese and western medicine. While taking a medication, attention should be paid to the side effects, and evaluate the progress of the adenomyosis. Therefore drug treatment and regular follow-up monitoring are important strategies. In this chapter, the mechanisms and side effects of common drug treatments for adenomyosis are introduced one by one.

10.1　Types and Options of Drug Therapy

10.1.1　Combined Oral Contraceptive (COC)

Combined oral contraceptives (COC) are a combination of steroid hormone preparations containing low doses of estrogen and progesterone. By inhibiting ovulation and endometrial growth, reducing menstrual flow and prostaglandin secretion [1], reducing uterine pressure and uterine spasm, and alleviating dysmenorrhea, COC is the first-line treatment for primary dysmenorrhea, endometriosis-related pain. It also can be used to treat adenomyosis-related pain and heavy menstrual bleeding. Either cyclic or continuous medication can be selected. Although COC is effective

J. Shi · Y. Dai · J. Leng (✉)
Department of Obstetrics and Gynecology, Peking Union Medical College Hospital,
Beijing, China

in treating endometriosis, the exact effect of dysmenorrhea and menorrhagia induced by adenomyosis has reported by little.

10.1.2 Progestins and Anti-Progestins

10.1.2.1 Levonorgestrel Intrauterine System (LNG-IUS)

Levonorgestrel intrauterine system (LNG-IUS) can continuously and slowly release levonorgestrel locally in the uterine cavity, causing a high-concentration progesterone environment in the uterine cavity, and down-regulating the estrogen and progesterone receptors. As a result, it has a significant inhibitory effect on prostaglandin synthesis in the endometrium, reducing intrauterine pressure and uterine contraction, relieving the severity of pain. LNG-IUS is not only suitable for contraception but also can treat dysmenorrhea and heavy menstruation and prevent recurrence after surgery. An observational study using LNG-IUS [2, 3] in 1100 gynecology patients with heavy bleeding and/or severe dysmenorrhea diagnosed with adenomyosis showed that LNG-IUS significantly reduced adenomyosis-related heavy menstrual periods and dysmenorrhea. The menstrual flow improvement reached a plateau stage after about 6 months and the relief of dysmenorrhea 1 year after placement. These symptom reliefs remained stable after 6 years of follow-up (all $p < 0.01$). Lin et al. 2018 studied the postoperative use of gonadotropin-releasing hormone analog (GnRH-a) ($n = 115$) followed with or without LNG-IUS; they showed that LNG-IUS was significantly better than the control group in improving pain and bleeding symptoms [4].

Youm et al. 2014 [5] studied the incidence of spontaneous expulsion of LNG-IUS among 481 women, and identified risk factors for the expulsion. They found that the incidence of expulsion rate was 7.9%, 9.1%, and 9.6% at 1, 2, and 3 years, respectively. The risk factors included adenomyosis, fibroids, heavy periods, dysmenorrhea, and prior treatment with GnRH-a. Li et al. 2016 [6] also studied the unplanned removal and shedding rates of LNG-IUS in patients with adenomyosis, compared with the normal population. The cumulative removal rate and shedding rate of LNG-IUS placed for 60 months were 9% and 16%, respectively. However, the reason for this high discontinued rate of LNG-IUS may be related to the enlargement of the uterine cavity, abnormal uterine contractility, and menorrhagia. Adequate information with the patients about this problem can help to improve collaboration [7]. Empirical treatment shows that for patients with uterine volume > 8 weeks, uterine cavity depth > 10 cm, and heavy menstrual flow causing anemia; GnRH-a can be used for 3–6 months to increase the continuation rate, but randomized controlled trial studies are lacking. Also, for patients with uterine cavity deformation, hysteroscopic-guided or ultrasound-guided placement can be considered, which can reduce the downward movement of LNG-IUS or even the fall off. For endometrial hyperplasia, combined with polyps, or small submucosal fibroids, hysteroscopy can be performed to remove these lesions and obtain the pathology before placing LNG-IUS.

10.1.3 Dienogest

The new progestogen (dienogest) has achieved good results in the treatment of endometriosis [8], inhibits ovulation, inhibits the growth of ectopic endometrium, alleviate dysmenorrhea, and reduce menstrual flow. A Phase III, randomized, double-blind, multicenter, placebo-controlled study on dienogest was completed in Japan in 2017 [9]. The study included 67 patients with dienogest treatment for 16 weeks. The pain in the treated group was significantly reduced compared with the placebo group and before treatment ($p < 0.01$). So far, in the study, patients had been taking continuous medication for more than 6 years and even after menopause as a long-term treatment. However, uterine bleeding is common during medication. About 20% of patients discontinued treatment, and the overall effect might be slightly worse than that of endometriosis treatment [10]. A study of 130 patients with adenomyosis [11] confirmed that the 2 mg/day dose of dienogest is effective and safe in treating adenomyosis.

10.1.4 Mifepristone

Mifepristone is an anti-progestin drug at the receptor level, without progesterone, estrogen, androgen, and anti-estrogen activities. Mifepristone has been approved for the treatment of uterine fibroids in China. The treatment of endometriosis and adenomyosis has not been approved by the China Food and Drug Administration (CFDA) and many countries. However, there have been many reports that mifepristone is safe and effective for treating adenomyosis for 3 months. Because mifepristone can cause estrogen to stimulate the endometrium continuously, the safety of long-term mifepristone treatment for more than 3 months on the endometrium has yet to be confirmed. Che et al. 2020 [12] found that mifepristone may effectively reduce the uterine volume and reduce the CA125 concentration by inhibiting the expression of CDK1 and CDK2, leaving the cells in a resting state and inducing apoptosis of endometrial epithelial cells.

10.2   Anti-Estrogen Drug

10.2.1 GnRH-a

GnRHa (Gonadotropin-releasing hormone agonist) is a class of synthetic GnRH derivatives that can compete with GnRH for the GnRH receptor. Continuous administration can down-regulate and change the effect of the GnRH receptor. It can inhibit the synthesis and release of LH (Luteinizing hormone) and FSH (follicle-stimulating hormone), thereby further inhibiting the synthesis of estrogen and progesterone in the ovaries, thus causing amenorrhea or to significantly reduce bleeding, relieve pain, and reduce uterine volume [13]. The dosage and precautions are the same as those for the treatment of endometriosis. The side effects are mainly perimenopausal symptoms caused by low estrogen levels, including bone calcium loss, etc., which can be treated by add-back [14]. There are flare-up effects after about 2 weeks of medication, some patients may have increased pain and excessive bleeding, etc., and they gradually disappear with the continuation of the drug. GnRH-a can reduce nitric oxide synthase levels to reduce endometrial free radical production, increase endometrial NK (natural killer) cell levels, and decrease interleukins 12, 15, and 18 [15]. Theoretically, GnRH-a pretreatment applied for 3–6 months before the assisted reproduction technique or the natural conception, can increase the chance of conception. GnRH-a is not only effective alone but is also often used as a preoperative pretreatment and postoperative consolidation treatment for patients with a large uterus or with anemia.

10.2.2 Aromatase Inhibitor

Aromatase (AR) is a complex enzyme of microsomal cytochrome P450. It composes of hemoglobin P450arom and reduced form of coenzyme NADPH and is widely expressed in the ovary. It is a key enzyme and rate-limiting enzyme that catalyzes the conversion of androgens to estrogen in the body. Aromatase inhibitor (AI) can specifically cause AR inactivation and inhibit estrogen production. Badawy et al. [16] performed a small randomized controlled clinical trial for the treatment of adenomyosis. It was found that letrozole (2.5 mg/d) was similar to goserelin in both symptom relief and uterine volume reduction, yet two patients were pregnant during a letrozole treatment. Besides, AIs have not been approved by the CFDA for the treatment of endometriosis and adenomyosis.

10.3 Androgenic Derivatives

Danazol and gestrinone are effective in treating endometriosis and can also relieve dysmenorrhea for adenomyosis. There were also reports of using danazol-containing IUDs to treat adenomyosis with significant results. Because of androgenic adverse reactions, danazol has been discontinued in China. However, it has been reported in the early years that the use of low-dose danazol at 100–200 mg/day can relieve dysmenorrhea of endometriosis or adenomyosis. Therefore, danazol has not been completely abandoned [17]. Gestrinone is an artificially synthesized triene 19-norsteroidal compound, which is an androgen derivative. It has strong anti-progestin and anti-estrogen activities and also has very weak estrogen and androgenic activities. By inhibiting the release of FSH and LH, it can directly act on eutopic and ectopic endometrial receptors, exert anti-progestin and anti-estrogen effects, increase free testosterone levels in the body, and reduce levels of sex hormone-binding globulin. It inhibits the growth of the endometrium and is used for the treatment of endometriosis and adenomyosis. The postoperative use of gestrinone in adenomyosis has a significant difference in menstrual volume, endometrial thickness, and dysmenorrhea score. However, irregular bleeding occurs during use, and the liver mainly metabolizes the drug so that long-term application may affect liver function [18].

10.4   Anti-Prostaglandin Drugs

There are currently no specific studies on non-steroidal anti-inflammatory drugs (NSAIDs) for the treatment of adenomyosis. The Cochrane systematic review (including 18 randomized controlled trials) reported that NSAIDs could reduce menstrual bleeding in 30% of patients, which was better than the placebo. Therefore NSAIDs can be used as a first-line drug for treating menstruation and relieve menstrual cramps. However, in about 18% of patients with dysmenorrhea, treatment with NSAIDs is ineffective [19]. To increase the effect of NSAIDs, they may be combined with COC. NSAIDs inhibit cyclooxygenase and reduce prostaglandin synthesis at the endometrial level, thereby alleviating dysmenorrhea and reducing menstrual bleeding (approximately 30%). There is no statistically significant difference in the efficacy of different types of NSAIDs while controlling menstrual-related anemia and pain without affecting fibroids or uterine size. Although NSAIDs can reduce uterine bleeding, they are less effective than other treatments, such as tranexamic acid or danazol and LNG-IUS. Patients with adenomyosis can use symptomatic treatment with NSAIDs when planning a pregnancy. NSAIDs commonly used in clinical practice include salicylic acid, paracetamol, indomethacin, ibuprofen, and mefenamic acid. All have fewer and mild adverse reactions and easily accepted by patients.

10.5   Hemostatic Drugs and Iron Supplements

Tranexamic acid is effective in treating heavy menstruation and may apply to adenomyosis with menorrhagia. However, there is no RCT study on its use to treat adenomyosis combined with menorrhagia. The usage is either oral or intravenous infusion. The patient should be monitored to reduce the possibility of thrombotic complications when using this product. For those with a tendency to thrombosis and myocardial infarction, it should be used with caution. For iron deficiency anemia, iron should be used at the same time to stop the bleeding, and vitamin C can increase the iron absorption rate.

10.6   Chinese Medicine and Herbs

Traditional Chinese medicine (TCM) is a great treasure of traditional medicine in China. It has its unique features in the understanding and treatment of adenomyosis. It is an understanding of Chinese medicine that the adenomyosis is related to "blood stasis." Its pathogenesis is due to external evil invasion, emotional trauma, physical factors, or surgical injury. The "menstrual blood" is due to retrograde blood stasis in the lower abdomen, which blocks the cells and causes disease. The treatment is based on promoting blood circulation and removing blood stasis, clearing away heat and removing toxic substances, and does not inhibit ovulation. There are many prescriptions of TCM for adenomyosis. Commonly used oral

Chinese herbs include Sanjie analgesic capsules, Guizhi Fuling capsules, and Shaofu Zhuyu decoction.

Wang et al. 2018 [20] and others searched 302 cases of adenomyosis treated with Chinese medicine in the literature and used the software "Traditional Chinese Medicine Assistance Platform" to enter 56 prescriptions for the treatment of adenomyosis. The highest frequency of herbs being used is the Angelica sinensis. This herb has actions to activate blood circulation, remove stagnation, and relieve pain; it corresponds to the core pathogenesis of dysmenorrhea and "blood stasis" in patients with adenomyosis. Besides, the use of enema to deliver Chinese herbal medicine is also practiced. As the female uterus is close to the rectum, it is the belief that the Chinese herbs can reach it, while avoiding the bitter taste aversion caused by oral herbs. Thus the Chinese patient is happy to accept. Jin et al. 2019 [21] treated 130 patients with adenomyosis with herbal enema and showed that the effective rate is 92.31%, which was higher than that of the mifepristone treatment group (76.92%), and the relapse rate and adverse reaction rate were low. In addition to oral and enema, acupuncture treatment can promote the operation of "qi" and the blood. Local warming and moxibustion can warm the meridians and reconcile "qi" and the blood.

Liu et al. 2018 [22] treated 30 adenomyosis patients with acupuncture combined with Chinese medicine. The main points of acupuncture are the uterus, Qihai, Zhongji, Hachiman, Shenshu, etc., once daily from 7 days before menstruation to the end of the menstruation, at the same time taking Yiqi analgesic decoction, 1 dose daily, for three consecutive menstrual cycles; the reported effective rate can reach 86.7%. The practice of Chinese medicine should not be just the use of Chinese herbs or a combination of herbs and western drugs. It should be the study of how to maximize the role of TCM and its combination of treatment to make the treatment of adenomyosis more effective, which are worthy of exploring. For the time being, there is still a long way to go before Chinese medicine can truly achieve both the symptoms of relief and the cure.

10.7   Combination of Treatments

10.7.1 The Combined Use of Drugs

The combined use of drugs includes the simultaneous use of two or more drugs, as well as the sequential use of several medications. Common drug combinations for adenomyosis include GnRH-a supplemented with OC (oral contraceptive)/LNG-IUS as a long-term treatment that can reduce the effects of a long-term low level of estrogen and consistent with health economics. The combined use of drugs helps to increase the continuation rate of LNG-IUS by reducing the uterine size and reduces the expulsion rate of the IUD (intra-uterine device). Also, the combination of TCM and western medicine is important combined drug therapy. Xuefu Zhuyu Capsule combined with LNG-IUS, Guizhi Fuling capsule combined with gestrinone, levonorgestrel combined with Sanjie analgesic capsule, etc. have been reported, with effects better than any single medication. However, attention must be paid to monitor the side effects and incompatibility of drugs when using different drugs together at the same time.

10.7.2 The Combined Use of Drugs and Surgery

In 2018, Rocha et al. [23] published a review that summarized a total of 16 studies in the past 7 years. The overall spontaneous pregnancy rate after conservative surgery was 18.2%. When supplemented with GnRH-a after surgery, the pregnancy rate can reach 40.7%, compared with only 15% of patients treated with supplements as a control group. However, there were also reports that the live birth rate of the combined drug and surgery group is not higher than that of the surgery only group. In a large-scale prospective study in 2009, Wang et al. [24] reported that for 114 patients with adenomyosis, GnRH-a was used for 6 months after conservative surgery. At 2 years follow up, there were 32 live births. However, this live birth rate was not higher than that of patients who underwent surgery alone. Some scholars conducted a follow-up study of 148 patients recurring laparotomy versus laparoscopy for severe diffuse adenomyosis for up to 6 years [25]. Regardless of the open surgery group or the laparoscopic surgery group, the postoperative GnRH-a + LNG-IUS/OC recurrence rate of symptoms was significantly lower than that of the single GnRH-a treatment group. Therefore, it is recommended for patients with conservative surgery to use GnRH-a for 4–6 months, which can inhibit the growth of residual lesions while waiting for the uterine incision to heal; it can also reduce the recurrence rate of pain. After that, those who have fertility demand should try to get pregnant, and those who have infertility problems should seek assisted reproductive technology, such as IVF (In vitro fertilization). For young patients without fertility requirements, contraceptive pills can be use instead, or LNG-IUS can be considered. Besides, preoperative GnRH-a can also increase hemoglobin concentration, reduce the size of the uterus, reduce the difficulty of surgical operation, and reduce anemia.

10.7.3 High-Intensity Focused Ultrasound (HIFU) and Drug Combination

The long-term management of HIFU treatment for adenomyosis in recent years has also been widely recognized. At present, the long-term management method commonly used after high-intensity focused ultrasound (HIFU) treatment of adenomyosis is mainly drug therapy, and related studies have confirmed that the long-term efficacy of HIFU combined with drugs for adenomyosis has significantly improved.

Guo et al. 2018 [26] retrospectively analyzed 78 patients with adenomyosis treated with HIFU, of which 45 patients were treated with HIFU only, 15 patients were treated with HIFU + LNG-IUS, and 18 patients were treated with HIFU + GnRH-a. At a 6-month and 12-month follow-up, the HIFU combined with GnRH-a and LNG-IUS groups improved significantly in terms of dysmenorrhea score, menstrual volume score, uterine size, and lesion size compared with the HIFU-treated group alone. Also, Ye et al. 2016 [27] retrospectively analyzed the efficacy of HIFU ablation alone, HIFU combined with GnRH-a or with LNG-IUS or with GnRH-a + LNG-IUS in the treatment of dysmenorrhea in adenomyosis; the combination therapy had significantly better relief than HIFU alone. Also, the recurrence rate was significantly reduced ($P < 0.008$).

There is no existing consensus for the indications and methods of combination therapy. From their clinical experience, Ye and Xu 2019 [28] summarized their recommended treatments for adenomyosis patients as follows: (a) If the patient's symptoms are mainly dysmenorrhea and the uterus size is <2 months of pregnancy, with no fertility demand, then the use of LNG-IUS on the first day after the end of the menstruation can be recommended; (b) For patients with uterine enlargement ≥2 months of pregnancy or increased menstrual flow and no fertility demand, GnRH-a is recommended for 4–6 months after HIFU treatment. Given the rapid recovery of uterine volume after GnRH-a, LNG-IUS was placed at 1 or 2 months before discontinuation of GnRH-a; (c) For patients with the significantly enlarged uterus and fertility demand, HIFU should be associated with GnRH-a treatment; then try to get pregnant as soon as possible after GnRH-a treatment, and if necessary, a short-term oral contraceptive before pregnancy can be used to control the recurrence.

To summarize, pharmacotherapy of adenomyosis is mainly applied to temporarily relieve pain, reduce bleeding, or reduce the size of lesions and the uterus. It is used for patients with mild to moderate symptoms or consolidates treatment to prevent a recurrence. Given the adverse reactions of drugs to varying degrees, they should be fully informed before treatment, and work out a treatment plan with the patient. During the medical treatment, patients should be monitored and followed up closely. For patients starting drug treatment, they should be followed up for 1–3 months to understand the occurrence of adverse reactions and deal with them accordingly. During the maintenance process, follow up every 3–6 months to understand the improvement of symptoms, such as bleeding, pain, and drug effects on the liver and kidney. For symptoms that do not improve or even progress, other treatments, such as surgery, should be considered.

References

1. Hauksson A, Ekström P, Juchnicka E, Laudanski T, Åkerlund M, Mats Åkerlund D. The influence of a combined oral contraceptive on uterine activity and reactivity to agonists in primary dysmenorrhea. Acta Obstet Gynecol Scand. 1989;68(1):31–4.
2. Li L, Leng JH, Dai Y, Zhang JJ, Jia SZ, Li XY, Shi JH, Zhang JR, Li T, Xu XX, Liu ZZ, You SS, Chang XY, Lang JH. The study LNG-IUS in the management of menorrhagia due to adenomyosis. Chinese Journal of Obstetrics and Gynecology. 2016;006:424–30.
3. Li L, Leng JH, Shi JH, Zhang JJ, Jia SZ, Li XY, Dai Y, Zhang JR, Li T, Xu XX. A prospective study of LNG-IUS for the treatment of severe dysmenorrhoea associated with adenomyosis. Chinese Journal of Obstetrics and Gynecology. 2016;005:345–51.
4. Lin CJ, Hsu TF, Chang YH, Huang BS, Jiang LY, Wang PH, Chen YJ. Postoperative maintenance levonorgestrel-releasing intrauterine system for symptomatic uterine adenomyoma. Taiwanese journal of obstetrics & gynecology. 2018;57(1):47–51.

5. Youm J, Lee HJ, Kim SK, Kim H, Jee BC. Factors affecting the spontaneous expulsion of the levonorgestrel-releasing intrauterine system. Int J Gynecol Obstet. 2014;126(2):165–9.
6. Li L, Leng JH, Jia SZ, Zhang JJ, Li XY, Shi JH. Analysis of the factors associated with unplanned removal and shedding of LNG-IUS in uterus with adenomyosis. Chinese Journal of Practical Gynecology and Obstetrics. 2016;32(11):1088–92.
7. Backman T, Huhtala S, Luoto R, Tuominen J, Rauramo I, Koskenvuo M. Advance information improves user satisfaction with the levonorgestrel intrauterine system. Obstet Gynecol. 2002;99(4):0–613.
8. Andres Mde P, Lopes LA, Baracat EC, Podgaec S. Dienogest in the treatment of endometriosis: systematic review. Arch Gynecol Obstet. 2015;292(3):523–9. Epub 2015/03/10. https://doi.org/10.1007/s00404-015-3681-6.
9. Osuga Y, Fujimoto-Okabe H, Hagino A. Evaluation of the efficacy and safety of dienogest in the treatment of painful symptoms in patients with adenomyosis: a randomized, double-blind, multicenter, placebo-controlled study. Fertil Steril. 2017;108(4):673–8.
10. Neriishi K, Hirata T, Fukuda S, Izumi G, Nakazawa A, Yamamoto N, Harada M, Hirota Y, Koga K, Wada-Hiraike O. Long-term dienogest administration in patients with symptomatic adenomyosis. J Obstet Gynaecol Res. 2018;44(8):1439–44.
11. Yu Q, Zhang S, Li H, Wang P, Zvolanek M, Ren X, Dong L, Lang J. Dienogest for Treatment of Endometriosis in Women: A 28-Week, Open-Label, Extension Study. Journal of women's health (Larchmt). 2019;28(2):170–7. Epub 2018/11/22. https://doi.org/10.1089/jwh.2018.7084. PubMed PMID: 30461337.
12. Che X, Wang J, He J, Yu Q, Sun W, Chen S, Zou G, Li T, Guo X, Zhang X. A new trick for an old dog: the application of mifepristone in the treatment of adenomyosis. J Cell Mol Med. 2019. Epub 2019/12/10; https://doi.org/10.1111/jcmm.14866.
13. Matsushima T, Akira S, Fukami T, Yoneyama K, Gynecology TTJ, Therapy MI. Efficacy of hormonal therapies for decreasing uterine volume in patients with Adenomyosis. Gynecol Minim Invasive Ther. 2018;7(3):119.
14. Wu D, Hu M, Hong L, Hong S, Ding W, Min J, Fang G, Guo W. Clinical efficacy of add-back therapy in treatment of endometriosis: a meta-analysis. Arch Gynecol Obstet. 2014;290(4):513–23.
15. Yang X, Huang R, Wang Y-f, Liang X-y. Pituitary suppression before frozen embryo transfer is beneficial for patients suffering from idiopathic repeated implantation failure. J Huazhong Univ Sci Tech. 2016;36(1):127–31. https://doi.org/10.1007/s11596-016-1554-2.
16. Badawy AM, Elnashar AM, Mosbah AA. Aromatase inhibitors or gonadotropin-releasing hormone agonists for the management of uterine adenomyosis: a randomized controlled trial. Acta Obstet Gynecol Scand. 2012;91(4):489–95.
17. Peng C, Zhou YF. A new exploration of the drug therapy of uterine adenopathy. China Family Planning and Obstetrics and Gynecology. 2019(4):18–20.
18. Duan H, Wang S, Hao M, Chen L, Tang J, Wang X, Peng YX, Zhang SC, Cao L, Yu JJ. Research of gestrinone-related abnormal uterine bleeding and the intervention in the treatment:a multicenter, randomized, controlled clinical trial. Chinese Journal of Obstetrics and Gynecology. 2016;2:98–102.
19. Oladosu FA, Tu FF, Hellman KM. Non-steroidal anti-inflammatory drug resistance in dysmenorrhea: epidemiology, causes, and treatment. Am J Obstet Gynecol. 2018;218(4):390–400. https://doi.org/10.1016/j.ajog.2017.08.108.
20. Wang LD, Leng JH, Zhang F, Li YN, Sun MX, Shi W, Xu L. Analysis and research on the law of chinese medicine for the treatment of uterine adenopathy based on the auxiliary platform of Traditional Chinese medicine. Shi Chen National Medcine 2018;29(3):742–4.
21. Jin Y, Liu ZK. Clinical observation of Traditional Chinese medicine enema for the treatment of adenomyosis. Journal of Practical Gynecologic Endocrinology 2019;6(2):72–7.
22. Liu AX, Huang WH, Lai CY. Acupuncture combined with Chinese medicine to treat 30 cases of uterine adenomyosis. Chinese Acupuncture & Moxibustion. 2018;38(6):655–6.
23. Rocha TP, Andres MP, Borrelli GM, Abrão MS. Fertility-sparing treatment of adenomyosis in patients with infertility: a systematic review of current options. Reprod Sci. 2018;25(4):480–6.

24. Ye MZ Deng XL, Zhu XG, Xue M. High-intensity focused ultrasound ablation combined GnRH-a and LNG-IUS in the treatment of uterine adenomyosis. Chinese Journal of Obstetrics and Gynecology. 2016;51(9):643–9.
25. Zhu L, Chen S, Che X, Xu P, Huang X, Zhang X. Comparisons of the efficacy and recurrence of adenomyomectomy for severe uterine diffuse adenomyosis via laparotomy versus laparoscopy: a long-term result in a single institution. J Pain Res. 2019;12:1917.
26. Guo Q, Xu F, Ding Z, Li P, Wang X, Gao B. High intensity focused ultrasound treatment of adenomyosis: a comparative study. Int J Hyperth. 2018;35(1):505–9.
27. Mingzhu Y,Xinliang D, Xiaogang Z, Min X. High-intensity focused ultrasound ablation combined GnRH-a and LNG-IUS in the treatment of uterine adenomyosis. Chinese J Obstet Gynecol. 2016;
28. Ye MZ, Xue M. Application of high-intensity focused ultrasound in the treatment of uterine adenopathy. Chinese Journal of Practical Gynaecology and Obstetrics. 2019;35(5):522–7.

The Surgical Treatment of Adenomyosis

11

Yi Dai and Jinhua Leng

Adenomyosis has a significantly negative impact on women's quality of life, causing abnormal uterine bleeding, dysmenorrhea, and chronic pelvic pain [1, 2]. Like endometriosis, adenomyosis is a benign disease, and although the definitive treatment of adenomyosis is hysterectomy, it is against many patients' desire to retain fertility. At present, there are currently no international guidelines to follow for either surgical or medical treatment for adenomyosis. But there is a growing consensus that adenomyosis needs long-term management plans, including pain and bleeding control, fertility preservation, and pregnancy assistance. In this context, the effect of conservative surgical treatment for long-term symptomatic relief, the benefit from the uterus-sparing surgery, and the pregnancy outcome after conservative surgery have become hot issues in the clinical treatment of adenomyosis. This chapter will discuss the surgical treatment of adenomyosis.

11.1 Indications of Surgery

The treatment of adenomyosis depends on the symptoms, severity, and fertility desire. Several medical treatments have been evaluated in adenomyosis, such as progestin [3], gonadotropin-releasing hormone agonists (GnRHa), nonsteroidal anti-inflammatory drugs (NSAIDs), levonorgestrel intrauterine system (LNG-IUS) [4], and combined oral contraceptives especially when used continuously [5]. These drug treatments are effective in reducing menstrual volume and pain in adenomyosis and are safe in long-term management. Therefore, the many experts' consensus in the diagnosis and treatment of adenomyosis agrees that we should give enough attempts to drug therapy before the decision of surgery.

Y. Dai · J. Leng (✉)
Department of Obstetrics and Gynecology, Peking Union Medical College Hospital, Beijing, China

© The Author(s), under exclusive license to Springer Nature Singapore Pte Ltd. 2021
M. Xue et al. (eds.), *Adenomyosis*, https://doi.org/10.1007/978-981-33-4095-4_11

Since in 1965, the first conservative surgical treatment for adenomyosis in young women was reported [6]; several new surgical methods for adenomyomectomy has been tried and reported. But the management of these women with adenomyosis-associated pain or subfertility is still highly controversial. So far we have not been able to reach a consensus on (a) who will definitively benefit from conservative surgery, (b) when is the appropriate time for patients to choose surgery, and (c) whether there will be an improvement in reproductive performance after the use of medical and/or surgical management. At present, the indications of surgery for adenomyosis should include (a) dysmenorrhea and hypermenorrhea that are difficult to control with medication and (b) intolerability or contraindications to long-term medication. For older patients who do not have fertility requirements, they can choose a total hysterectomy; for younger patients who desire to preserve fertility or the uterus, they can select conservative surgery, that is, fertility-sparing operations. For patients undergoing conservative surgery, they should be fully informed of the possibility of recurrence of symptoms, because the uterus is preserved.

11.2   Preoperative Assessment

The preoperative evaluation of adenomyosis should first summarize the symptoms, previous treatment, and its results, to judge the indication and timing of the operation.

11.2.1 Age

Age should be an important factor to consider before surgery, especially before the decision-making of patients with adenomyosis associated infertility, because it might be the most critical factor of fertility. It is well-known that fertility declines after 35 years of age, and the chance of miscarriage increases [7].

11.2.2 Infertility

For every patient, detailed medical history should be inquired, including years of infertility, clinical symptoms, diagnosis, and previous medical and surgical treatment, as well as whether there is a history of repeated abortion or repeated embryo transfer failure. At the same time, we should carefully check whether the patients have the previous diagnosis of pelvic endometriosis, myoma, endometrial polyp, hydrosalpinx, etc. The ovulation function (combined with menstrual history, B-ultrasonic monitoring, and urine LH measurement) and the ovarian function (age, Antral Follicle Count (AFC), Anti-Mullerian Hormone (AMH), and basic endocrine) also should be evaluated in patients complaining of infertility. Other auxiliary examinations, if indicated, can also include hysteroscopy, CA125, MRI, and semen analysis. The evaluation of ovarian reserve function is very important. In the case of basic follicle stimulating hormone (FSH) is more than 12 IU/L, and ultrasonography shows that bilateral Antral Follicle Count Score (AFCS) is less than 5, and/or AMH is less than 1.1 ng/ml, the ovarian reserve function failure can be considered.

Therefore, the surgical plan for patients with adenomyosis and infertility problem should insist that the gynecologist and the reproductive medicine specialist, if possible, cooperate to jointly develop a treatment plan for the patient, rather than the unilateral decision of the gynecologist.

11.2.3 Laboratory Examinations

Preoperative laboratory examination and evaluation includes routine blood tests and CA125 measurements. For patients with moderate anemia before surgery, pretreatment before surgery to correct anemia will improve the safety of surgery and help patients to recover quickly after surgery. GnRHa is a drug commonly used before the operation for uterine adenomyosis, which can correct anemia and reduce the uterine volume. Usually, three monthly GnRHa injections can be given before surgery. Preoperative anemia can also be improved through supportive treatment, such as iron supplements.

11.2.4 Preoperative Imaging

The preoperative imaging of adenomyosis is more important than the preoperative diagnosis. It can help to predict the operation approach, the effectiveness of the operation, and the risk of the surgery.

11.2.5 Preoperative Pelvic Ultrasound Evaluation

Pelvic ultrasound examination is the most commonly used auxiliary examination before adenomyosis surgery, and it is also the preferred imaging examination [8, 9]. A recent meta-analysis has shown that the sensitivity and specificity of 2D transvaginal ultrasound scanning (TVUS) to diagnose adenomyosis was 83.8% and 63.9%, while the sensitivity and specificity of 3D TVUS are 88.9% and 56.0% [10], respectively. Not only the rate of diagnosis of adenomyosis is high, but ultrasound is also the basis for the classification of adenomyosis [11, 12]. Symptoms of uterine motility detected during an ultrasound scan also help predict the condition during the operation. A negative uterine motility sign indicates that adenomyosis may involve the uterine serosa with adhesion to surrounding organs (such as the bowels). The assessment of whether the disease is accompanied by deep invasive endometriosis at the same time has a reference effect on the choice of laparoscopic or open surgery before surgery.

Some ultrasound diagnosticians have put forward an ultrasonic report system of adenomyosis, aiming to report the ultrasonic results of adenomyosis more regularly and systematically. A new reporting system for adenomyosis was proposed by

Van den Bosch et al. 2019 [11] which described the location of the adenomyosis, into anterior, posterior, left, right, and fundus, and the involvement <25%, 25%–50%, and > 50% of uterine volume and the size of adenomyosis. The scoring system can provide a more detailed ultrasound description of the adenomyosis image. However, other scholars have proposed a definition of adenomyosis severity scoring system [13]. Tellum et al., 2018 [14] also developed a clinical prediction model that uses the most relevant features, like myometrial cysts, fan-shaped echo, hyperechoic islets, globular uterus, thickness/thinnest ratio, etc., to identify the disease. These ultrasound-based assessment systems not only help to standardize the ultrasound description of adenomyosis but also provide a better assessment of the severity of adenomyosis before surgery and the prediction of improved fertility outcomes after surgery. They also make it easy for preoperative preparation and communication with patients. However, these models currently require external validation and more evidence to support its reliability. Such verification requires the joint participation of clinical gynecologists, ultrasound doctors, obstetricians, and reproductive medicine doctors, which will be worthwhile for us to work in this direction in the future.

11.3   Preoperative MRI Evaluation

Because of its advantages of intuitive images, not operator dependence, multi-parameter imaging, and multi-planar imaging, MRI is increasingly applied for preoperative evaluation of uterine adenomyosis [15]. At this time, the information provided by MRI is not only a diagnosis of adenomyosis but also offers detailed information for surgery. For example, MRI can give a more precious classification to refine the surgical treatment of different adenomyosis. In the previous chapter on diagnosis, the imaging-clinical classification based on MRI appearance has been described. The four subtypes proposed by Kishi et al. 2012 [12] and the complex 11 subtypes from A to K proposed by Bazot et al. 2018 [16] are conducted under the guidance of imaging experts. We need to further correlate these subtypes with clinically effective treatment outcomes, especially the improvement of symptoms after uterine-sparing surgery and the relationship between pregnancy outcomes of infertile patients and different types of adenomyosis.

Besides, MRI can still provide additional details about the preoperative evaluation of adenomyosis. For example, on the T2-weighted MRI, there are multiple spot-like high signals in the muscle layer. These spot-like high signals correspond to histopathological endometrial tissue with hyperplasia, with or without changes in the bleeding. The surrounding low-signal area corresponds to smooth muscle hyperplasia of the myometrium [17]. Small endometrial cysts can also be found, which are very helpful for the localization of preoperative adenomyomas (see Fig. 11.1). The T1-weighted sequence also helps identify high-signal-intensity lesions [18] that represent bleeding areas, with a positive predictive value of 95% [19]. The detection of these adenomyosis lesions before surgery is very instructive to detect and define the lesions as much as possible and reduce residual lesions after surgery.

Fig. 11.1 Adenomyosis of
the posterior uterine wall
with cystic changes
(reproduced with
permission from reference)

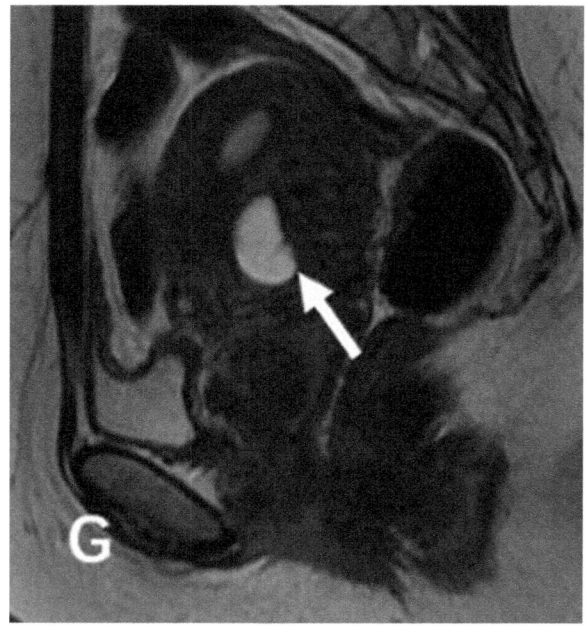

MRI can also be used to determine the presence or absence of intrapelvic endometriosis before surgery, especially deep infiltrates lesions. A typical example is the
"hourglass sign." Local fibrous tissue hyperplasia in the posterior cervix or vagino-
rectal endometriosis leads to adhesion of surrounding structures, partial or complete
closure of the uterine rectal fossa, thickening of the uterine and sacral ligaments,
and invasion of the rectum causing teardrop-like traction and forward involving the
uterine serosa layer (Fig. 11.2), leading to external adenomyoma, resulting in a classic "hourglass"-like appearance. This sign indicates severe adhesion of the posterior
pelvic cavity and may be combined with deep infiltrating endometriosis of the
uterosacral ligaments and the pouch of Douglas. The evaluation of these imaging
details before surgery has important reference and significance for judging the difficulty of operation, choosing an open or laparoscopic approach, and also involving
rigorous preoperative bowel preparation.

11.4   Surgical Treatment

11.4.1   Total Hysterectomy

Total hysterectomy is a radical cure for adenomyosis and the gold standard for
treating patients without fertility requirements. After a hysterectomy, there is theoretically no chance of recurrence. Hysterectomy can be performed by abdominal,
vaginal, or laparoscopic approaches. In recent years, it can also be a single-port
laparoscopic [20, 21] and transvaginal natural orifice transluminal endoscopic

Fig. 11.2 External
adenomyosis shows the
hourglass sign (reproduced
with permission from
reference)

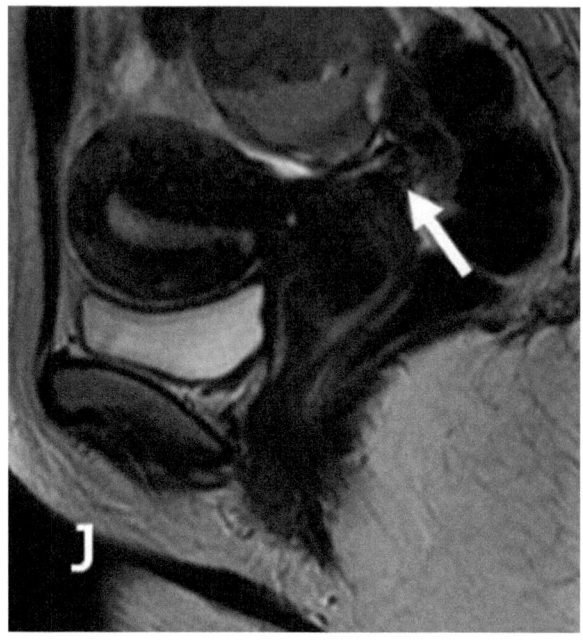

assisted hysterectomy [22]. It must be emphasized that subtotal hysterectomy should be avoided, and there have been more cases of continuous vaginal bleeding after hysterectomy [23], recurrent dysmenorrhea, and occurrence of the cervical stump or recto-vaginal adenomyosis. This management of these conditions can be tricky. Patients may need to have repeated medical treatment. Residual cervical resection is accompanied by an increased risk of bladder and rectal injury. Cochrane's analysis also found no evidence that subtotal hysterectomy is superior to total hysterectomy in reducing pelvic support disorders or decreased sexual function [24].

For different surgical approaches, minimally invasive surgery is preferable to traditional open surgery from the perspective of doctors or patients. Transvaginal hysterectomy is also a safe option for patients without severe pelvic adhesions [25] and have good postoperative results. Clinical studies report that laparoscopic surgery does not appear to increase the risk of perioperative complications. Single-port laparoscopy, which has started in recent years, is also safe, without increasing the rate of laparotomy or risk of complications [26]. It should also be noted that adenomyosis is often associated with pelvic endometriosis and may be accompanied by complicated pelvic deep-infiltrating endometriosis lesions, including recto-vaginal endometriosis nodule and complete obliteration of recto-vaginal fossa.

In the study of the risk factors of laparoscopic hysterectomy, some researchers have reported that type II adenomyosis is one of the independent high-risk factors for laparoscopic hysterectomy [27]. In an early comparative study of the complications of vaginal hysterectomy in patients with adenomyosis or uterine fibroids, the adenomyosis group had an increased risk of bladder injury during surgery [28]. Therefore, a total hysterectomy for adenomyosis can be a difficult hysterectomy. The transabdominal hysterectomy is still a relatively safe procedure in patients with adenomyosis with severe pelvic adhesions and deeply infiltrating endometriosis (DIE).

There are a few specific comparative studies on the prognosis of patients with a total hysterectomy. Total hysterectomy obviously can permanently resolve the complications of abnormal uterine bleeding. As for pain-related symptoms, total hysterectomy also works well. It is possible that in patients with endometriosis, there is a risk of recurrence of symptoms after uterine removal alone. However, in a recent prospective study, laparoscopic hysterectomy for premenopausal women with cyclic pelvic pain associated with endometriosis, the satisfaction index after hysterectomy remained high [29]. Therefore, the use of hysterectomy for patients with adenomyosis can be confirmed.

11.5   Conservative Surgery

From the perspective of alleviating symptoms and promoting fertility, patients with adenomyosis should initially choose drug treatment. For patients of reproductive age who cannot tolerate long-term drug treatment or failed drug treatment, they have fertility requirements or need to retain the uterus. Surgery is fertility-sparing procedures.

The purpose of conservative surgery is to remove the adenomyosis lesion, preserve the uterus, and even preserve fertility. Conservative surgery for adenomyosis was reported in 1965 [30]. Before the 1970s, the most common suture materials were silk and gut, which could lead to strong foreign body reactions after surgery, increasing complications, such as suture failure. Despite this, surgical resection of adenomyoma continues to improve. Furthermore, the development of absorbable sutures has significantly reduced severe tissue reactions. The development of energy devices, such as electric, ultrasonic, and high-frequency scalpels, has reduced intraoperative bleeding and improved surgical safety. But today, conservative surgery compared with total hysterectomy remains a challenge for gynecologists and patients. There are, however, still authors who believe that the uterus-sparing surgery [31] or fertility-sparing surgery cannot be considered a standard treatment for adenomyosis [1]. The reason is that (a) although the existing clinically reported procedures are effective in improving symptoms, no standard procedure has yet been established. When the literature is reviewed, a total of 2365 cases of adenomyosis resection were reported from 1990 to 2018, of which Japanese scholars reported 2123 (89.8%). It can be seen that the validity of regional clinical studies is relatively limited, and more extensive clinical data are needed. Therefore international studies are required to verify problems associated with multiple interventions in conservative surgery [31]. (b) Due to the infiltration pattern and unclear border of adenomyosis, no surgical technique can guarantee the complete removal of the adenomyosis lesions from the uterine myometrium. (c) Any conservative procedure will damage the healthy uterine muscle, and it will increase the risk of uterine rupture and placental implantation during pregnancy.

11.5.1 Types of Conservative Surgeries for Adenomyosis

Conservative surgery for adenomyosis is divided into (a) adenomyomectomy for focal adenomyosis (1), (b) cytoreductive surgery for diffuse adenomyosis, and (c) endometrial ablation or resection for intrinsic adenomyosis.

11.5.2 Adenomyomectomy

There have been reports of various surgical approaches involving laparotomy and laparoscopic and robotic adenomyoma resections [32–34]. Adenomyoma resection includes wedge resection of adenomyoma and resection of cystic adenomyoma. Wedge resection was to remove part of the myometrium and its underlying adenomyosis. In this procedure, the wound cavity after resection is relatively small, and some adenomyoma tissue will remain on one or both sides of the incision. The wound of the uterine wall is repaired by suturing the remaining muscular layer with the serosa. According to the tension of the wound wall of the muscular wall, the suture method can be a continuous suture, interrupted suture, or U-type reduction suture reinforcement (see Fig. 11.3) [35] and muscle layer overlap suture to fill the wound cavity [36].

11.5.3 Cytoreductive Surgery for Diffuse Adenomyosis

Focal debulking of diffuse adenomyosis is based on a new concept completely different from traditional surgical methods. This surgical technique mainly includes two parts: (a) try to remove the lesions of the muscular layer and (b) repair the huge defect of the uterine wall and reconstruct the uterine wall, which is called "uterine reconstruction," and establish the endometrium with a different technique. The methods of constructing the muscle flap and the myometrial muscle flap are slightly different, and their purposes are to repair a large defect of the uterine wall and reconstruct the uterus. This procedure is mainly used in diffuse adenomyosis and

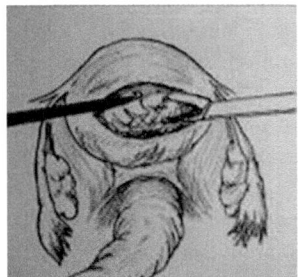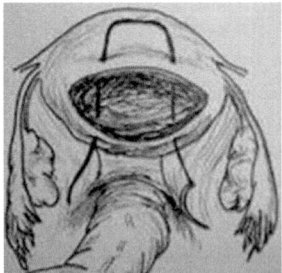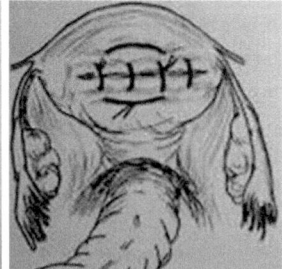

Fig. 11.3 shows U-shaped reduction suture reinforcement to close the wound cavity of the uterine wall. (reproduced with permission from Sun et al. 2011, Chinese medical journal)

severe adenomyosis. Different scholars have reported different techniques for excision and uterine reconstruction. Japanese scholars have made significant contributions to this technique, and they have explored many different methods of resection and reconstruction. The incision on the uterine wall can be vertical, diagonal, and H-shaped incisions [37, 38]. Uterine reconstruction methods include U-shaped sutures, "overlapping flaps," "triple flaps," and so on. In order to delay or reduce the postoperative recurrence in these procedures, it is necessary to remove as many adenomyosis lesions as possible, and they are likely to enter the uterine cavity. It is more difficult to remodel the uterine muscle wall after the adenomyosis lesions are removed. Therefore open abdominal surgery is easier to perform than this procedure.

11.5.4 Symptom Relief After Conservative Surgery

In terms of the improvement of symptoms and infertility, the efficacy of conservative surgery is positive. The smaller the remaining lesion, the more successful the symptom relief is. A systematic literature review published in 2014 [31] included 64 studies and 1049 patients who underwent conservative surgery for symptomatic adenomyosis. After complete excision of adenomyosis, the postoperative dysmenorrhea response rate was 82.0%, the menstrual period reduction response rate was 68.8%, the pregnancy rate was 60.5%, postoperative remission rate of dysmenorrhea was 81.8%, the menstrual reduction rate was 50.0%, and the pregnancy rate was 46.9%. Younes and Tulandi, 2018 [39] also confirmed that after conservative surgery, over three-fourths of women would experience symptom relief; on the other hand, the pregnancy rates varied widely with or without adjuvant medical treatment. The conservative surgery can be comparable with drug treatment in terms of symptom relief and pregnancy rate during postoperative follow-up.

11.5.5 Recurrence of Symptoms After Conservative Surgery

Surgery is effective in relieving symptoms; however, the recurrence of symptoms after surgery reflects the two sides of a problem. Relapse is due to the presence of residual adenomyosis tissue. Unlike uterine fibroids, the boundary between adenomyosis lesions and the normal myometrium is not clear, and the lesion is difficult to remove completely. This is the main reason for pain recurrence after conservative surgery, and it has a certain correlation with the size of residual lesions [35].

11.5.6 Uterine Rupture After Conservative Surgery

Symptom relief, recurrence, fertility outcomes, and risk of uterine rupture after uterine-preserving surgery are issues that should be addressed. Osada et al. 2018 [1] reviewed a total of 2365 cases of adenomyoma resection reported since 1990, including 2123 (89.8%) in Japan. In a total of 397 postoperative pregnancies, there were 337 (84.89%) live births and 23 uterine ruptures. A meta-research showed that the highest pregnancy rates were reported after resection of cystic adenomyosis and focal adenomyosis, having a higher pregnancy rate than diffuse adenomyosis and lower uterine rupture rates [2, 40]. The risk of uterine rupture (6.8%) after conservative surgery for adenomyosis is much higher than that for uterine fibroid removal (about 0.26%) [1, 41]. This point should be taken seriously by all surgeons who undergo conservative surgery for adenomyosis.

For conservative surgery for adenomyosis, it is important to maintain the firmness of the uterine wall. Otsubo et al. 2016 [42] used MRI and/or ultrasonography to examine the thickness of the uterine wall before pregnancy in women undergoing conservative surgery for diffuse adenomyosis. As a result, 10 of the 23 women had premature births, and 13 had continued pregnancy. The uterine rupture occurred in two cases of abortion. They found that the thickness of the uterine wall is related to the risk of uterine rupture during pregnancy. The optimal uterine wall thickness before pregnancy should be between 9 and 15 mm to reduce the risk of uterine rupture during pregnancy. Morimatsu et al. 2007 [43] reported a case of pregnancy that occurred 1 month after conservative surgery, and the uterine rupture occurred after 28 weeks of gestation. Kodama et al. 2015 [44] reported the results of 71 cases of laparoscopic adenomyoma resection, including one case of uterine rupture, which was pregnancy at 4 months after surgery.

Wound healing is usually a complex process involving inflammation, angiogenesis, new tissue formation, and tissue remodeling. After myomectomy or cesarean section, the uterine rupture in the scar area is usually manifested by abnormally high collagen concentration in the uterine muscle wall tissue near the ruptured site, and smooth muscle fibers are reduced, so the tension of the uterine muscle layer is damaged [45]. Cold knife, scissors, etc. are commonly used in open surgery for conservative adenomyosis operation, while electrosurgical equipment, such as monopolar electric diathermy and laser knife, is commonly used in laparoscopy. Although energical equipment can reduce the bleeding and speeds up the procedure, yet, it also can cause thermal injury at the incision wound in the muscular layer, resulting in poor healing of the incised tissue. As a result, there are many cases of tissue fibrosis at the uterine boundary between the abnormal tissue and normal tissue. Histological studies have shown that thermal injury had greatly affected the wound healing, which can lead to suture failure, because tissue necrosis, scarring, and excessive collagen deposition increase the risk of wound dehiscence.

The adverse effect of any thermal injury on wound healing is even more detrimental in the healing wounds after adenomyosis surgery. An analysis of 23 cases of uterine rupture after conservative surgery for adenomyosis, 15 patients had surgery using monopolar cautery, high-frequency electrosurgery, laser knife, and other high-energy instruments; two cases used monopolar electrosurgery knife. The remaining six patients did not have information on the type of intraoperative cutting instruments used. There have been no reports of uterine rupture due to the use of a scalpel. Therefore, there seems to be a clear link between uterine rupture and the use of high-energy power instruments. Thus, if the safety of laparoscopic and open conservative surgery in terms of uterine rupture and technical difficulty are to be compared, laparoscopic surgery with its use of high-energy thermal devices may increase the risk of uterine rupture during pregnancy [46, 47].

To summarize the possible risk factors for uterine rupture after conservative surgery of adenomyosis, it may include: the electrosurgical instruments used (such as cold knife or energy device), the amount of adenomyosis removed, the extent and size of uterine muscle defects, the uterine reconstruction technique, wound hematoma and infection, contraceptive time, and the surgical procedure. Besides, there are reports of high-risk pregnancy, such as placental implantation after adenomyosis surgery. Therefore, the consensus of experts on adenomyosis recommends a detailed communication of the pros and cons and possible risks of conservative surgery for the adenomyosis. From the safety and technical perspective of facilitating the removal of the adenomyosis and repairing the uterine muscle layer, open surgery is even more suitable.

11.6 Conservative Surgery Improves Adenomyosis-Related Infertility

There is currently insufficient evidence to support the benefits of conservative surgery to improve the adenomyosis-related infertility. Kishi et al. 2014 [48], however, reported that in 102 women who wished to become pregnant, the total clinical pregnancy rate was 31.4% (32/102) after conservative surgery. When grouped by age (under 40 and above 40), the clinical pregnancy rates were 41.3% and 3.7%, respectively. Of the six patients in the >40-year-old group, five had abortions. Therefore, this study showed that in women over 40 years of age, the benefits of surgery were not obvious.

Although surgery is not recommended as a first-line treatment for the treatment of adenomyosis with infertility, conservative surgery is recommended for patients with severe symptoms or failure of repeated assisted reproductive assistance [49]. If the patient is unwilling to receive assisted reproductive assistance after surgery, spontaneous natural pregnancy after GnRHa treatment can be attempted.

11.7 Conclusion

Treatment of adenomyosis is quite complex and controversial. Although hysterectomy is still the ultimate treatment for women with severe symptoms, conservative surgical options should be offered for women who wish to maintain fertility. Conservative surgery can improve symptoms associated with clinical treatment. In patients with adenomyosis, conservative surgery can be an option when clinical treatment fails. Obstetric complications after extensive uterine reconstruction can increase, such as uterine rupture, placental implantation, placenta previa, etc. These complications should be paid attention to and fully discussed with patients before surgery. At present, there are many conservative surgical procedures, and there is still a lack of standardized surgical procedures. Data supporting the effectiveness of these surgical procedures are still limited, and further elaborate clinical studies are needed.

References

1. Osada H. Uterine adenomyosis and adenomyoma: the surgical approach. Fertil Steril. 2018;109(3):406–17.
2. Oliveira MAP, et al. Surgery in adenomyosis. Arch Gynecol Obstet. 2018;297(3):581–9.
3. Osuga Y, Watanabe M, Hagino A. Long-term use of dienogest in the treatment of painful symptoms in adenomyosis. J Obstet Gynaecol Res. 2017;43(9):1441–8.
4. Li L, et al. Treatment of symptomatic adenomyosis with the levonorgestrel-releasing intrauterine system. Int J Gynaecol Obstet. 2019;146(3):357–63.
5. Pontis A, et al. Adenomyosis: a systematic review of medical treatment. Gynecol Endocrinol. 2016;32(9):696–700.
6. Van Praagh I. Conservative surgical treatment for adenomyosis uteri in young women: local excision and metroplasty. Can Med Assoc J. 1965;93(22):1174–5.
7. Rocha TP, et al. Fertility-sparing treatment of Adenomyosis in patients with infertility: a systematic review of current options. Reprod Sci. 2018;25(4):480–6.
8. Cunningham RK, et al. Adenomyosis: a sonographic diagnosis. Radiographics. 2018;38(5):1576–89.
9. Sam M, et al. Accuracy of findings in the diagnosis of uterine adenomyosis on ultrasound. Abdominal Radiology. 2020;45(3):842–50.
10. Andres MP, et al. Transvaginal ultrasound for the diagnosis of adenomyosis: systematic review and meta-analysis. J Minim Invasive Gynecol. 2018;25(2):257–64.
11. Van den Bosch T, et al. Sonographic classification and reporting system for diagnosing adenomyosis. Ultrasound Obstet Gynecol. 2019;53(5):576–82.
12. Kishi Y, et al. Four subtypes of adenomyosis assessed by magnetic resonance imaging and their specification. Am J Obstet Gynecol. 2012;207(2):114–e1-114. e7.
13. Lazzeri L, et al. A sonographic classification of adenomyosis: interobserver reproducibility in the evaluation of type and degree of the myometrial involvement. Fertil Steril. 2018;110(6):1154–1161. e3.
14. Tellum T, et al. Development of a clinical prediction model for diagnosing adenomyosis. Fertil Steril. 2018;110(5):957–964.e3.
15. Champaneria R, et al. Ultrasound scan and magnetic resonance imaging for the diagnosis of adenomyosis: systematic review comparing test accuracy. Acta Obstet Gynecol Scand. 2010;89(11):1374–84.
16. Bazot M, Daraï E. Role of transvaginal sonography and magnetic resonance imaging in the diagnosis of uterine adenomyosis. Fertil Steril. 2018;109(3):389–97.
17. Kroencke TJ. MRI for diagnosis of adenomyosis: unsung and underutilized. Gynecol Obstet Investig. 2005;60(3):154.
18. Agostinho L, et al. MRI for adenomyosis: a pictorial review. Insights Imaging. 2017;8(6):549–56.
19. Bazot M, et al. Ultrasonography compared with magnetic resonance imaging for the diagnosis of adenomyosis: correlation with histopathology. Hum Reprod. 2001;16(11):2427–33.
20. Lee J, et al. Single-port access versus conventional multi-port access total laparoscopic hysterectomy for very large uterus. Obstet Gynecol Sci. 2015;58(3):239–45.
21. Song T, et al. Single port access laparoscopic-assisted vaginal hysterectomy for large uterus weighing exceeding 500 grams: technique and initial report. J Minim Invasive Gynecol. 2010;17(4):456–60.
22. Baekelandt J, et al. Hysterectomy by transvaginal natural orifice transluminal endoscopic surgery versus laparoscopy as a day-care procedure: a randomised controlled trial. BJOG Int J Obstet Gynaecol. 2019;126(1):105–13.
23. Sasaki KJ, et al. Persistent bleeding after laparoscopic supracervical hysterectomy. JSLS: J Soc Laparoendoscopic Surg. 2014;18(4)
24. Sokol AI, Green IC. Laparoscopic hysterectomy. Clin Obstet Gynecol. 2009;52(3):304–12.
25. Pepas L, Deguara C, Davis C. Update on the surgical management of adenomyosis. Curr Opin Obstet Gynecol. 2012;24(4):259–64.

26. Kim SH, et al. Postoperative outcomes of natural orifice transluminal endoscopic surgery-assisted vaginal hysterectomy and conventional laparoscopic-assisted vaginal hysterectomy: a comparative study. Obstet Gynecol Sci. 2018;61(2):261–6.
27. Saito A, et al. Preoperative assessment of factors associated with difficulty in performing total laparoscopic hysterectomy. J Obstet Gynaecol Res. 2017;43(2):320–9.
28. Furuhashi M, et al. Comparison of complications of vaginal hysterectomy in patients with leiomyomas and in patients with adenomyosis. Arch Gynecol Obstet. 1998;262(1–2):69–73.
29. Berner E, et al. Pelvic pain and patient satisfaction after laparoscopic supracervical hysterectomy: prospective trial. J Minim Invasive Gynecol. 2014;21(3):406–11.
30. Van Praagh I. Conservative surgical treatment for adenomyosis uteri in young women: local excision and metroplasty. Can Med Assoc J. 1965;93(22):1174.
31. Grimbizis GF, Mikos T, Tarlatzis B. Uterus-sparing operative treatment for adenomyosis. Fertil Steril. 2014;101(2):472–487.e8.
32. Chung Y-J, et al. Robot-assisted laparoscopic adenomyomectomy for patients who want to preserve fertility. Yonsei Med J. 2016;57(6):1531–4.
33. Shim JI, et al. A comparison of surgical outcomes between robot and laparoscopy-assisted adenomyomectomy. Medicine. 2019;98(18).
34. Chong GO, et al. Long-term efficacy of laparoscopic or robotic adenomyomectomy with or without medical treatment for severely symptomatic adenomyosis. Gynecol Obstet Investig. 2016;81(4):346–52.
35. Ai-jun S, et al. Characteristics and efficacy of modified adenomyomectomy in the treatment of uterine adenomyoma. Chin Med J. 2011;124(9):1322–6.
36. Takeuchi H, et al. Laparoscopic adenomyomectomy and hysteroplasty: a novel method. J Minim Invasive Gynecol. 2006;13(2):150–4.
37. Fujishita A, et al. Modified reduction surgery for adenomyosis. Gynecol Obstet Investig. 2004;57(3):132–8.
38. Saremi A, et al. Treatment of adenomyomectomy in women with severe uterine adenomyosis using a novel technique. Reprod Biomed Online. 2014;28(6):753–60.
39. Younes G, Tulandi T. Conservative surgery for adenomyosis and results: a systematic review. J Minim Invasive Gynecol. 2018;25(2):265–76.
40. Tan J, et al. Reproductive outcomes after fertility-sparing surgery for focal and diffuse adenomyosis: a systematic review. J Minim Invasive Gynecol. 2018;25(4):608–21.
41. Sizzi O, et al. Italian multicenter study on complications of laparoscopic myomectomy. J Minim Invasive Gynecol. 2007;14(4):453–62.
42. Otsubo Y, et al. Association of uterine wall thickness with pregnancy outcome following uterine-sparing surgery for diffuse uterine adenomyosis. Aust N Z J Obstet Gynaecol. 2016;56(1):88–91.
43. Morimatsu Y, et al. Uterine rupture during pregnancy soon after a laparoscopic adenomyomectomy. Reproductive Med Biol. 2007;6(3):175–7.
44. Kodama K, et al. Fukukukyoka-shikyusenkinsho-tekishutsujutsu go ni shikyuharetsu, yuchakutaiban wo mitome shikyutekishutsu ni itatta ichi-shorei.[a case of hysterectomy due to uterine rupture and placenta accreta after laparoscopic adenomyomectomy.]. J Jpn Soc Endometriosis. 2015;36:189–92.
45. Pollio F, et al. Uterine dehiscence in term pregnant patients with one previous cesarean delivery: growth factor immunoexpression and collagen content in the scarred lower uterine segment. Am J Obstet Gynecol. 2006;194(2):527–34.
46. Chao A-S, et al. Laparoscopic uterine surgery as a risk factor for uterine rupture during pregnancy. PLoS One. 2018;13(5)
47. Parker WH, et al. Risk factors for uterine rupture after laparoscopic myomectomy. J Minim Invasive Gynecol. 2010;17(5):551–4.
48. Kishi Y, Yabuta M, Taniguchi F. Who will benefit from uterus-sparing surgery in adenomyosis-associated subfertility? Fertil Steril. 2014;102(3):802–807.e1.
49. Dueholm M. Uterine adenomyosis and infertility, review of reproductive outcome after in vitro fertilization and surgery. Acta Obstet Gynecol Scand. 2017;96(6):715–26.

Uterine Artery Embolization Treatment for Adenomyosis

12

Zhiwen Fan

For symptomatic patients with adenomyosis, a variety of treatment options are available based on the patient's age, physical and psychological needs, and traditional treatment methods. These treatments include surgical removal, subtotal hysterectomy, or total hysterectomy. However, the surgical removal of adenomyosis is difficult and not satisfactory for diffuse adenomyosis; thus, it is not often performed. Adenomyosis also increasingly begins at a younger age of onset, and there is a need to retain the uterus. In addition to the above surgical treatment, oral contraceptives, Mirena (LNG-IUS), gonadotropin-releasing hormone agonist (GnRH-a), and other conservative treatments are also options for managing adenomyosis. The poor compliance of long-term oral contraceptives, the irregular vaginal bleeding after LNG-IUS, and menopausal symptoms of the expensive GnRH-a contribute to the short-term use of these methods. Therefore, for patients who require treatment for their symptoms, but unwilling to undergo surgical treatment because they are afraid of surgery or have other reasons not to undergo surgery (such as medical and surgical contraindications or religious beliefs), there is a choice of uterine artery embolization (UAE) method. This interventional embolization technology has a history of nearly 20 years and has achieved satisfactory clinical efficacy [1]. Its advantages are the preservation of the uterus, easy operation, quick recovery after surgery, and few postoperative complications. Therefore it has become one of the effective alternatives in the treatment of symptomatic adenomyosis.

Z. Fan (✉)
Department of Gynecology and Obstetrics, Third Xiangya Hospital of Central South University, Changsha, Hunan, China

12.1   The Principle of UAE Treatment of Adenomyosis

Adenomyosis is the invasion of the glandular into the uterine myometrium from the basal layer of the endometrium, causing diffuse or focal hyperplasia of the surrounding smooth muscle and fibrous connective tissue. These lesions have a rich neovascular network and poor tolerance to ischemia and hypoxia. However, the surrounding normal uterine tissue has a rich vascular communication network and a strong tolerance to ischemia and hypoxia. Therefore after bilateral uterine arteries are embolized, the vascular network and the blood supply to the adenomyosis are blocked. Thus it can result in ischemic necrosis of the lesion, which will then be dissolved and absorbed. Finally, the adenomyosis reduces in sizes or even disappears. In term, it can effectively reduce the amount of menstrual bleeding, to achieve the purpose of relieving the heavy bleeding.

12.2   Indications and Contraindications of UAE

12.2.1 Indications of UAE

1. The patient is willing to receive UAE treatment and understand the possible complications.
2. Symptomatic adenomyosis without fertility requirements, including dysmenorrhea and excessive menstruation.
3. Patients with adenomyosis who have failed non-surgical treatment, refused surgery, or have multiple previous surgeries, which are difficult to achieve a good result in repeat surgical treatment.
4. Patients with pelvic endometriosis (including ovarian endometriosis cysts) should be informed that UAE is not effective for the above diseases. If the patient fully understands and requests, UAE can be used to treat uterine adenomyosis, combined with laparoscopic treatment of pelvic endometriosis (including ovarian endometrioma).
5. For patients with symptomatic adenomyosis with fertility requirements, the use of UAE should be with caution; if patients strongly require UAE treatment, they must be informed that UAE may cause ovarian or endometrial necrosis, resulting in secondary infertility. Even though it is rare, it may still happen.
6. In patients with recurrence of adenomyosis after UAE, 3-D digital CT angiography may indicate that the blocked uterine artery has been reopened. If the blood supply of the lesion does not come from the ovarian source, the patient may undergo a second UAE treatment.

12.2.2 The Contraindications for UAE [2]

1. Complicated urogenital system infection.
2. Coexistence of known or suspected gynecological malignancies.

3. General contraindications for interventional embolization, such as a recent history of stroke, contrast agent allergy, skin infection at the puncture point, renal insufficiency, or severe immune suppression of the body.
4. Digital 3-D reconstruction by CT angiography suggests that the blood supply of the adenomyosis lesions is mainly from bilateral ovarian arteries.

12.3   Preoperative Assessment and Examination

1. Medical history and evaluation: A patient for UAE surgery needs a comprehensive evaluation, including a detailed gynecological history, such as menstrual history, previous pregnancy, birth planning, gynecological diseases, and previous pelvic surgery, and medical history to identify various comorbidities, such as diabetes, high blood pressure, taking anticoagulants, etc. It is necessary to fully inform the patient and sign the informed consent of the operation for her to understand the advantages and disadvantages of the UAE treatment, the expected effect, and potential complications.
2. Evaluation of dysmenorrhea:The visual analog scale (VAS) of pain and chronic pain rating scale are used to evaluate the degree of dysmenorrhea in patients with adenomyosis. The VAS pain score is mainly a score for the patient's last dysmenorrhea. The chronic pain rating scale is mainly used to score the degree of dysmenorrhea in the past 6 months and its impact on life and daily activities [3].
3. Evaluation of menstrual flow: Heavy menstrual flow refers to menstrual volume > 80 ml per cycle (equivalent to more than 20 sanitary napkins). Scanty menstrual flow refers to menstrual volume < 5 ml per cycle (less than one sanitary napkin).
4. In addition to routine examinations, such as blood routine, coagulation function, liver and kidney function, and electrocardiogram, it is recommended that patients undergo sex hormone level testing on days two to four before menstruation to assess ovarian function. Blood levels of CA125 are recommended before and after treatment. Before surgery, for patients with the large uterus (such as more than 3 months of pregnancy) or medical complications, such as obesity, diabetes, and hypertension, if any of them is at risk of thrombosis, it is recommended to perform a Doppler venous ultrasound examination of both lower extremities to assess the presence or absence of thrombosis before surgery.
5. Imaging assessment: MRI examination is currently the most accurate assessment method. MRI examination can provide better spatial resolution and contrast resolution and is not affected by sound and shadow. It can accurately assess the size, location, and number of lesions. It can be used as one of the effective differential diagnosis methods of adenomyosis and uterine fibroids [4, 5]. Ultrasound examination is an acceptable alternative method, which has the advantage of being cheap. Depending on the size of the uterus, transabdominal and transvaginal B-ultrasound examinations are sometimes required for evaluation. CT can clearly show the condition of pelvic blood vessels at all levels. Compared with

the invasiveness and lag of digital subtraction angiography (DSA), CT angiography combined with digital 3-D reconstruction technology can evaluate the source of the blood supply artery of adenomyosis before operation to plan the surgical approach and reduce the blindness of the operation, which can improve the success rate of the operation [6, 7]. It can also effectively classify the type of blood supply to the adenomyosis:

Based on the degree of bilateral uterine artery blood supply to the adenomyosis, it is divided into (a) bilateral balanced type of uterine artery blood supply, (b) unilateral main type of uterine artery blood supply, and (c) only one side uterine artery blood supply.

Based on the degree of vascularization of the lesion, the lesion is divided into (a) rich blood flow type, (b) general blood flow type, and (c) non-rich blood flow type or scanty blood flow type.

According to the above characteristics of blood supply, the selection, distribution, and quantification of the embolic agent specifications can be guided to fully embolize the vascular network of the adenomyosis lesion. Therefore, assessing whether the blood supply of adenomyosis lesion is abundant and the source of blood supply to the adenomyosis before surgery, one can predict the efficacy of UAE treatment of adenomyosis. It is recommended that qualified hospitals perform digital 3-D reconstruction of CT angiography before UAE to clarify the blood supply artery and blood supply type of adenomyosis lesions to assist in screening patients suitable for UAE and guide the operation [8].

12.4   Operation Procedure of UAE

After the successful arterial puncture procedure, arteriography is performed first to determine the structure and distribution of the abdominal pelvic blood vessels and to assess the vascular network and to see whether there is a variation in the blood supply to the lesion.

1. The choice of embolizing agent: UAE can choose from many embolizing agents. Generally, granular embolizing agents are selected. They can be divided into absorbable and non-absorbable. The absorbable embolizing agent is sodium alginate microsphere particles (KMG), and the non-absorbable embolic agent is represented by polyvinyl alcohol (PVA). The other embolic agents commonly used for other organs, such as steel rings, absolute ethanol, and ultra-liquid lipiodol, are not recommended for use in UAE. The choice of the particle size of the embolizing agent: the particle diameter of the embolizing agent is mainly 500–700 µm, and some can also be selected from 300–500 µm or 700–900 µm. In adenomyosis, the internal vascular network is relatively small, and the outer vascular network is not obvious. In order to achieve a better embolization effect, a smaller particle embolization agent can be appropriately selected. The effect of arterial embolization is inversely proportional to the particle size of the embolizing agent.

2. Degree of embolism: Embolism is divided into two types: complete embolism and incomplete embolism. Incomplete embolism is based on blocking as much of the vascular network of the lesion as possible, without embolizing the normal vascular network of the uterus. The CT DSA imaging will show a complete or partial disappearance of the vascular network of the adenomyosis. The complete embolization requires that as much as possible, the embolization agent is released into the uterine artery and its branches that supply blood to the adenomyosis and the vascular network of the adenomyosis to be all blocked. In DSA, the imaging showed that the vascularity of the adenomyosis is completely disappeared, and the main uterine artery only partially appears or not appear at all. In order to obtain better clinical efficacy, adenomyosis must be a complete embolism.

3. Intraoperative medication: Patients with adenomyosis may also have associated with hidden endometritis due to long-term menorrhagia. Therefore, antibiotics may be used to prevent infection in UAE surgery when it is necessary.

12.5   Postoperative Treatment of UAE

The arterial puncture point can be compressed to stop the bleeding, and the puncture point can be bandaged with elastic tape, and the lower extremity must be immobilized for 6–12 hours; if a blood vessel clip is used, the immobilization duration can be shortened, and the patient can get out of the bed earlier. Observe the color and skin temperature of both lower extremities after the operation, and mark the pulsating of the dorsal arteries of the foot. Observe regularly to prevent thrombosis. Postoperative antibiotics are not routinely used.

12.6   Complications of UAE

1. Intraoperative complications:
   (a) Local bleeding or hematoma: Hemorrhage or hematoma at the puncture site is a relatively common complication, mostly manifested as subcutaneous swelling at the puncture site, but severe cases can cause a large pelvic retroperitoneal hematoma. After the elimination of coagulation defects before surgery, it can be treated by compression and hemostasis.
   (b) Arterial spasm: During the operation, the guidewire repeatedly stimulates the blood vessel, especially in a long operation, which may cause arterial spasm, resulting in leg numbness and pain during the operation, and it will then affect the operation. Analgesic drugs can be used to relieve pain, and intra-arterial injection of 2% lidocaine 5 ml is used to reduce the pain stimulation at the wound.
   (c) Arterial puncture injury: Arterial puncture injury during operation is rare. However, because the pelvic artery is located in the retroperitoneal space, once the artery is punctured, it will be difficult to compress it for hemostasis, resulting in a large retroperitoneal hematoma. The bleeding will threaten the

life of the patient; an emergency laparotomy is needed to stop the bleeding. Therefore, the UAE procedure should be performed with care and gentleness, and the direction of the blood vessel path should be recognized, following the direction of no or minimal resistance when resistance is encountered.

2. Postoperative complications:

    (a) Pain: Almost all patients will experience pain after surgery. It is currently believed that pain is related to ischemia of the adenomyosis lesion and the uterus after UAE. The degree of pain varies from mild to severe colic. The analgesic method depends on the severity of the pain, and non-steroidal anti-inflammatory drugs, self-controlled analgesia, and opioids orally or parenterally can be selected. The duration of the pain varies, and it is gradually relieved 2–5 days after surgery. If the pain is more than 1 week and is more severe, alert should be raised to the possibility of serious complications, such as secondary infection and accidental thrombosis.

    (b) Post-embolism syndrome: Post-embolism syndrome manifests as pelvic pain, nausea, vomiting, fever, fatigue, myalgia, discomfort, and leukocytosis. Most occurred within 24 hours after surgery and gradually improved within 7 days. It is a common postoperative complication. Postoperative fever is generally not higher than 38 °C, as postoperative heat absorption usually does not require antibiotic treatment.

    (c) Thrombosis: it is divided into arterial and venous thrombosis. Arterial thrombosis is mainly caused by excessive compression of the puncture point or embolization by the embolization agent, etc., which causes ischemic necrosis of tissues, organs, and limbs. Prompt discovery is especially important, and pulsations of the dorsalis pedis artery should be monitored every 30 minutes after surgery. If there is thrombosis or embolism, it is necessary to balance the risk of thrombolysis and secondary bleeding. Relevant departments in the hospital should be consulted and prepare for thrombus removal. Venous thrombosis mostly forms in the lower limb, and it occurs after postoperative immobilization of the legs or bed rest. The presentation is manifested as lower limb swelling, skin color changes, and skin temperature changes; after thrombosis, if emboli fall off, which can lead to serious life-threatening complications, such as pulmonary embolism and cerebral embolism, resuscitation needs to be urgently available.

    (d) Arterial rupture or dissection: As a serious complication, surgical repair is required.

    (e) Mis-embolized other blood vessels: Because the anterior branch of the internal iliac artery not only branch out the uterine artery, it also has the vesical artery, vaginal artery, internal pudendal arteries, etc. When other pelvic arteries are mistakenly embolized, large and small labial necrosis, bladder necrosis, and other complications may occur.

    (f) Infection: The operation of UAE involves only a type I incision. Wound infection is relatively rare. Inflammation is mainly due to necrosis of the lesion after embolization, resulting in aseptic inflammation. However, the infection can be due to communication between the uterine cavity and the outside world via the cervix and vagina. Poor hygienic care can cause uterine cavity infection, leading to endometritis, pyometra, salpingitis, tubal ovarian abscess, or secondary infection of the lesion. At this time, antibiotic treatment is often effective. If it is necessary, surgical drainage or uterine excision is required, and in severe cases, fatal sepsis can occur. The long-term sequel of infection may also result in intrauterine adhesions and infertility.

(g) Allergic reaction or rash: anti-allergic treatment may be given.

(h) Vaginal discharge: Some patients will have persistent vaginal bloody discharge after surgery, usually within 2 weeks, and very few may last for several months. Short-term vaginal discharge is common.

(i) Menorrhagia: Some patients have partial endometrial necrosis after embolization of the uterine artery vascular network, and there may be a significant decrease in menstrual flow, but no obvious hormonal abnormalities are seen. If there are no fertility requirements, follow up observation is not necessary.

(j) Amenorrhea: a long-term complication of UAE is treatment-induced amenorrhea. Ovarian amenorrhea is mainly due to the cessation of blood supply to the ovary, because sometimes the uterine artery gives rise to an ovarian branch in which blood flow is blocked by UAE, resulting in ischemic necrosis of the ovary, ovarian failure, and amenorrhea. Long-term hormone replacement therapy may be required to maintain the level of hormones in the body. Uterine amenorrhea is caused by extensive ischemic necrosis of the endometrium, and the growth of the endometrium is impaired. It does not affect hormone secretion and can be observed, but the patient may have a fertility problem.

(k) Others: Other serious complications are rare. The incidence of venous thromboembolic complications is about 0.4%. There are also fatal sepses associated with UAE operations, including femoral nerve injury, bilateral iliac artery embolism, ischemic uterine infarction, large and small labial necrosis, local bladder necrosis, bladder and uterine fistula, uterine wall injury, embolism agent spillage leading to both toes, or even rare complications, such as necrosis of the heel. About 2.4%–3.5% of patients need to be admitted to the hospital again, and 1.0%–2.5% of patients need unplanned surgery. However, overall, UAE mortality has not increased compared with hysterectomy [1].

12.7 Follow-Up Time and Efficacy Evaluation after UAE Treatment

1. Follow-up time: After UAE treatment, re-evaluation is required at 1, 3, and 6 months and once a year after that. The contents of the follow-up include changes in the size of the lesion, menstrual conditions, sex hormone levels, and changes in dysmenorrhea and CA125 levels.

2. Evaluation of clinical efficacy: A large number of clinical trial data showed that 98%–100% of patients could tolerate and complete the operation, 85%–94% of patients had improved abnormal vaginal bleeding, and 77%–79% of patients got improvement in dysmenorrhea, and the average uterine volume decreased by 35%–60%. For patients who were followed up for more than 5 years, more than 75% of patients had normal or improved menstrual flow after the operation. The cumulative recurrence rate at 5 years was 10%–15%, which was lower than the recurrence rate of surgical removal. About 20% of patients may require further surgery after UAE, such as hysterectomy, removal of residual adenomyosis, or UAE again, to control the symptoms of adenomyosis.

12.8   Other Issues

1. Effect on ovarian function: It is currently believed that whether the ovarian function is affected is positively related to age. The prevalence of early menopause after UAE for women aged 45 and younger is 2%–3%, while the incidence for women older than 45 can reach 8%. It is considered that the embolization agent enters the ovarian artery along with the blood flow to reduce the ovarian function [9].
2. Pregnancy after UAE: At present, there is no definite conclusion about the safety of pregnancy after the UAE. There are reports of cases of successful pregnancy after UAE and delivery. However, adverse outcomes of pregnancy after UAE, including spontaneous abortion, premature delivery, abnormal placenta, pre-eclampsia, postpartum hemorrhage, etc., have also been observed, and the rate of cesarean section has also increased. Among them, some of the increased risks are related to the high proportion of women in UAE who are elderly and infertile. In addition, hysteroscopy examination of patients 3–9 months after UAE found that only 40.2% of patients after the UAE had a normal endometrial appearance. Therefore UAE may cause endometrial abnormality that affects pregnancy and its outcomes. Therefore, for women considering future births, UAE should be used with caution in the treatment of adenomyosis [1].
3. Repeat UAE treatment can be performed, but the evidence for these operations is limited. Available data show that 1.8% of patients received UAE treatment again. If the choice is appropriate, 90% of patients can successfully control symptoms after the second UAE operation. Therefore, for patients with recurrent adenomyosis after UAE, it is recommended to perform CT angiography followed by digital 3-D reconstruction to assess the condition of the pelvic vascular network, especially whether the uterine artery is recanalized or whether there are other new blood vessels to supply blood to the lesion to assess whether UAE can be effectively repeated.

References

1. de Bruijn AM, et al. Uterine artery embolization for the treatment of adenomyosis: a systematic review and meta-analysis. J Vasc Interv Radiol. 2017;28(12):1629–1642. e1.
2. Keung JJ, Spies JB, Caridi TM. Uterine artery embolization: a review of current concepts. Best Pract Res Clin Obstet Gynaecol. 2018;46:66–73.
3. Von Korff M, et al. Grading the severity of chronic pain. Pain. 1992;50(2):133–49.
4. Deshmukh SP, et al. Role of MR imaging of uterine leiomyomas before and after embolization. Radiographics. 2012;32(6):E251–81.
5. Chapron C, et al. Relationship between the magnetic resonance imaging appearance of adenomyosis and endometriosis phenotypes. Hum Reprod. 2017;32(7):1393–401.
6. Liu Ruilei DE, Chunlin C, Ping L. The construction of digital three-dimensional model of the pelvic and abdominal pelvic artery vascular network and its application in the uterine arterial embolism entrance planning. Chinese Journal of Obstetrics and Gynecology. 2014;002:89–93.
7. Chen Chunlin CL, Lei T, Ping L, Jianxuan L, Bin C, Hui D, Jun W. The digital three-dimensional model of the abdominal pelvic vascular guides the selection of intravascular intervention intubation. Chinese Journal of cardiovascular diseases. 2015;24(3):252–6.
8. Jiang Bingyang LP. The choice of 3D reconstruction technology and individual treatment options for uterine adenomyosis. Chinese Journal of Practical Gynaecology and Obstetrics. 2017;33(2):141–5.
9. Worthington-Kirsch R, et al. The Fibroid registry for outcomes data (FIBROID) for uterine embolization: short-term outcomes. Obstet Gynecol. 2005;106(1):52–9.

Principles and Protocols of HIFU Ablation for Adenomyosis

13

Xiaogang Zhu, Min Xue, and Felix Wong

13.1 The Principles of HIFU Treatment

Selective ablation of endometriotic lesions in the myometrium reduces the extent and sizes of adenomyosis lesions and limits the ectopic endometrial functions and growth. Eventually, it may achieve the purpose of improving symptoms.

13.1.1 Indications

The indications of high-intensity focused ultrasound (HIFU) ablation for adenomyosis are (a) symptomatic adenomyosis with a single-layer uterine wall thickness ≥ 30 mm, (b) clinically diagnosed adenomyosis (clinical manifestation + US/MRI), (c) no history of radiotherapy in the lower abdomen, (d) no contraindications for sedation and analgesia during HIFU ablation, and 5) rule out pain symptoms mainly due to pelvic endometriosis.

13.1.2 HIFU Ablation Procedure

The operation procedure is the same as that of HIFU ablation to uterine fibroids [1]. The patient needs to be positioned and prepared before treatment. Under sedation

X. Zhu · M. Xue
Department of Gynecology and Obstetrics, Third Xiangya Hospital of Central South University, Changsha, Hunan, China

F. Wong (✉)
School of Women's and Children's Health, The University of New South Wales, Sydney, NSW, Australia
e-mail: fwong3@hotmail.com.hk

© The Author(s), under exclusive license to Springer Nature Singapore Pte Ltd. 2021   123
M. Xue et al. (eds.), *Adenomyosis*, https://doi.org/10.1007/978-981-33-4095-4_13

and analgesia and real-time image monitoring, point-line-surface combined scanning and ablation is used to complete the treatment at each layer, until the completion of HIFU ablation can be achieved [1]. The treatment range would be (a) symmetric diffuse type, if the thickness of the anterior and posterior uterine walls exceeds 30 mm, both front and back walls need to be ablated; (b) asymmetric diffuse type, only ablate the uterine wall with a thickness of more than 30 mm; and (c) focal type, only ablate the focal lesions.

Because the structure of adenomyosis is completely different from that of fibroids and the boundary is unclear, that is, there is no pseudocapsular interface, the ultrasonic energy deposition and diffusion are different and more difficult, and the required treatment dose is significantly increased by about 20–30%. At the same time, the apparent grayscale change appears later than that of fibroids; the dose distribution has to be uniform when the grayscale change does not appear. The average energy power is preferably at 400 W.

13.1.3 Matters That Need Attention During HIFU Ablation

1. The extent of treatment: Adenomyosis is a solid tumor. The purpose of treatment is to improve the clinical symptoms caused by adenomyosis. The boundary between adenomyosis and the surrounding myometrium is unclear, so the treatment extent cannot include all the lesions. Under safe conditions, as much ablation of the adenomyosis lesion as possible should be performed; that will relate to the degree of symptom improvement and duration of relief.
2. Treatment tolerance: Patients with adenomyosis have a high local prostaglandin level in the lesion, which is related to her severe pelvic pain or dysmenorrhea. The more severe the symptoms of dysmenorrhea, the more obvious the pain response during treatment. The use of intravenous dexamethasone and analgesic can greatly improve pain tolerance during HIFU ablation for adenomyosis.
3. Ultrasound dosage: The energy deposition and heat diffusion in adenomyosis are more difficult than uterine fibroids. Therefore, the dose and adverse reactions may increase. Because the adenomyosis has no pseudocapsule, the energy diffusion is easy to spread. It is then necessary to keep a safe distance from the uterine serosa (at least about 1–1.5 cm) during the ablation procedure, to avoid heat from reaching and breaking through the serosa and causing damage to surrounding tissues and organs, such as the bladder, and intestinal injury.
4. The protection of the endometrium: Adenomyosis is of irregular shape and size; therefore, the HIFU ablation areas can be irregular and unpredictable. Besides, the endometrium of patients with adenomyosis often has old surgical scars, which are easy to allow the deposition of ultrasound energy leading to endometrial damage. Thus HIFU procedure should take cautions to avoid damage to the endometrium, particularly for those who wish to have children. Informing patients of the pros and cons and possible risks in detail before HIFU treatment is important. During the HIFU ablation, maintain a safe distance of at least 1.5 cm between the target focal point and the endometrium and try to choose a

spot treatment to avoid accumulating at one focal point of too much energy that may diffuse unpredictably and damage the endometrium. Only doctors with experience should operate HIFU ablation for adenomyosis. Special attention to the protection of the endometrium is to protect the fertility of the patient as much as possible.

13.1.4 Importance to Communication with Patients

1. Despite the special nature of the adenomyosis, the difficulty of its ablation, and the extent of ablation, most patients can obtain a good ablation effect. However, a few patients may require multiple treatments or repeat treatment. If the HIFU ablation fails to give the desired result, we shall tell the patients that it is necessary to combine drugs or utilize LNG-IUS and other long term management to delay postoperative recurrence.
2. Usually, after the ablation effect is achieved, the symptoms are often relieved or disappeared. Yet, in some patients, there may be no change in the symptoms, which may be related to some associated endometriosis in the pelvis. Although doctors can try to rule out pelvic endometriosis by various non-invasive tests, some endometriosis still cannot be detected. Invasive procedures, like laparoscopy or open surgery, are the only confirmative investigations for suspected pelvic endometriosis.
3. Due to the presence of abnormal nerves in the adenomyosis lesion, the pain or discomfort of the patient during ablation can be more obvious, similar to the pain symptoms during normal menstruation. Although there will be some pain relief after the analgesic and sedative drugs given during the HIFU ablation, it cannot be completely eliminated. Therefore patients need to have psychological preparation before the treatment and managed as discussed previously.
4. The purpose of ultrasound ablation therapy is to relieve or reduce symptoms. Changes in the size of the uterus and the lesion due to reabsorption of the ablated tissue are secondary. Although they will reduce in sizes after HIFU ablation, some may not.
5. After HIFU ablation, the necrosis and aseptic inflammation of the adenomyosis are more irritating to the uterus; thus, the patient's pain response can be more severe. The duration may last for 6–12 hours postoperatively. It is necessary to pay attention to the treatment of postoperative pain in patients after HIFU treatment. If necessary, low-dose dexamethasone and oral analgesics are given to relieve these post-HIFU painful symptoms.

13.1.5 Clinical Effect

According to the enhanced MRI evaluation, almost all patients with adenomyosis can have regular or irregular ablation of adenomyosis, which is related to the shape of the lesion. After HIFU ablation, about 80%–90% of patients can get different degrees of symptom relief, of which in about 90% of patients, symptom relief occurs during the first menstrual cycle, and others require three menstrual cycles. The 2-year follow-up results showed that 13% of patients relapsed after remission of symptoms, usually within 1 year. Patients who have their symptoms relapse can be treated with HIFU ablation again. However, it should be noted that patients with associated pelvic endometriosis may not have obvious symptom relief after treatment, or they can have pain relapse quickly.

13.2 HIFU Treatment Protocol for Adenomyosis

1. HIFU alone: It is a single HIFU ablation treatment. It requires no auxiliary therapy before and after the ablation, because HIFU is not a radical treatment for adenomyosis. When patients begin to have their first menstruation after HIFU ablation, symptoms of adenomyosis may recur; even though the overall effective rate of HIFU treatment is 70%–90% [1–3]. Ultrasound-guided HIFU is an effective treatment for both focal and diffuse adenomyosis lesions; Zhang et al. 2014 [2] showed that complete relief of dysmenorrhea at the 3 months follow-up was significantly higher among women with focal adenomyosis than among those with diffuse adenomyosis. However, with the accumulation of clinical experience, the application of a single HIFU treatment has gradually decreased because of the increase in recurrence after a longer follow-up period.

2. First HIFU + GnRH-a: Combined with GnRH-a (3–6 monthly injections) after HIFU, this condition is mainly used for patients with large uterine volume. Simply HIFU treatment alone cannot completely ablate all adenomyosis lesions, and any remaining adenomyosis may continue to grow. Combined with GnRH-a after HIFU ablation is to inhibit the growth and recurrence of residual lesions. It is especially suitable for patients who have fertility requirements after surgery. After HIFU ablates most of the adenomyosis, GnRH-a continues to suppress the residual lesions, improve the uterine environment, and increase the ability of uterine pregnancy. Besides, for patients with heavy menstrual flow as the main symptom, the uterine volume is still large after HIFU ablation, before the adenomyosis begins its absorption and volume reduction. Therefore, combined GnRH-a treatment during this period is also a very good indication to reduce the menstrual flow. However, the combined GnRH-a treatment after surgery may increase the financial burden of patients because of the expensive medication.

3. First GnRH-a + HIFU: 3–6 monthly injections of GnRH-a treatment are given before HIFU ablation. GnRH-a can improve the patients' menstrual flow and anemia and reduce the volume of uterine and adenomyosis lesions, the vascularity of the adenomyosis, and the HIFU ablation time, and facilitate the HIFU treatment. Therefore pre-operative GnRH-a treatment is especially indicated for patients with heavy menstrual volume, severe anemia, large uterine volume, and abundant vascular supply to the adenomyosis. If necessary, some patients can still have combined GnRH-a for further treatment after surgery [4]. In general,

the combined use before and after surgery is generally recommended not to exceed 6 months in total, to avoid GnRH-a-related side effects.

4. First HIFU + LNG-IUS: After HIFU ablation to control the symptoms and ablated the lesions, for patients with small to normal uterine volume, the placement of an LNG-IUS in the uterus helps to delay the appearance of dysmenorrhea, reduces menstrual flow, and reduces the recurrence of adenomyosis. It is suitable for patients with no fertility requirements after surgery. Some research results show that comparing the effects of HIFU treatment alone, HIFU combined with LNG-IUS treatment, HIFU combined with GnRH-a treatment of adenomyosis, the latter two methods are significantly better than HIFU treatment alone. Their recurrence rates are significantly reduced [5].

5. HIFU + GnRH-a + LNG-IUS: Combined with GnRH-a (3–6 months) after HIFU, then LNG-IUS is inserted 3 months after GnRH-a is completed. This combined treatment is mainly used for patients with large uterine volume or heavy in menstrual flow but without fertility demand. Recent studies had confirmed this comprehensive combination treatment effectively provides long-term management for adenomyosis, significantly reduce dysmenorrhea or menstrual flow [4, 6].

References

1. Zhou M, Chen JY, Tang LD, Chen WZ, Wang ZB. Ultrasound-guided high-intensity focused ultrasound ablation for adenomyosis: the clinical experience of a single center. Fertil Steril. 2011;95:900–5.
2. Zhang X, Li K, Xie B, He M, He J, Zhang L. Effective ablation therapy of adenomyosis with ultrasound-guided high-intensity focused ultrasound. Int J Gynaecol Obstet. 2014;124:207–11.
3. Cheung VY. Current status of high-intensity focused ultrasound for the management of uterine adenomyosis. Ultrasonography. 2017;36(2):95.
4. Yang X, Xiaofei Z, Lin B, et al. Combined therapeutic effects of HIFU, GnRH-a and LNG-IUS for the treatment of severe adenomyosis. Int J Hyperth. 2019;36:486–92.
5. Guo Q, et al. High intensity focused ultrasound treatment of adenomyosis: a comparative study. Int J Hyperth. 2018;35(1):505–9.
6. Ye M, et al. Clinical study of high intensity focused ultrasound ablation combined with GnRH-a and LNG-IUS for the treatment of adenomyosis. Zhonghua Fu Chan Ke Za Zhi. 2016;51(9):643–9.

HIFU Ablation

14

Xiaogang Zhu, Felix Wong, and Min Xue

Ultrasound monitoring is the method to apply diagnostic imaging technology to guide the treatment of high-intensity focused ultrasound (HIFU). The treatment is called ultrasound-guided HIFU (USgHIFU) ablation surgery. Compared with focused ultrasound ablation surgery guided by magnetic resonance (MRgHIFU), HIFU under ultrasound monitoring is less expensive. Besides, ultrasound monitoring can also provide real-time image monitoring of changes in uterine position and bowel movement during the ablation procedure. The therapeutic effect can be shown by the gray-scale changes at the target lesions during HIFU ablation. Under ultrasound monitoring, all these gray-scale changes, absence of Doppler blood flow, and non-perfusion of ultrasound contrast agent at the adenomyosis lesion will indicate the effects of HIFU; thus, it is a reliable monitoring indicator [1]. In addition, ultrasound monitoring is quieter, and patients do not need to be in a relatively enclosed treatment environment, like in an MRI room. Therefore we are illustrating the use of a USgHIFU ablation system, which is more popular in China. In this chapter, we will introduce the preoperative preparation and the therapeutic process of focused ultrasound ablation surgery for adenomyosis.

X. Zhu · M. Xue
Department of Gynecology and Obstetrics, Third Xiangya Hospital of Central South University, Changsha, Hunan, China

F. Wong (✉)
School of Women's and Children's Health, The University of New South Wales, Sydney, NSW, Australia
e-mail: fwong3@hotmail.com.hk

14.1 USgHIFU Treatment Procedure

14.1.1 Preoperative Preparation

(a) Ultrasound simulation assessment: Before surgery, the patient should have a simulation assessment on the ultrasound treatment system, to determine whether the ultrasound energy pathway, i.e., the acoustic pathway, is safe, whether the lesion can be displayed, and whether the target focus can reach the lesion; for patients with IUDs, they should have the IUD removed. Patients should have finished their menses and have no vaginal bleeding before the HIFU ablation. At the time of the assessment test, the patient needs to be able to retain her urine and tolerate a large bladder volume. Routine blood investigations include liver and kidney functions, complete blood count, and coagulation profile, and, if necessary, the pregnancy test, Pap smear (TCT), and high vaginal swab culture are performed. For patients with hypertension or with a history of chest pain, chest X-ray and an electrocardiogram are done to assess their cardiovascular condition. Finally, a pelvic MRI examination before the assessment should be available to assess the adenomyosis lesion in detail, and the MRI image can be incorporated into the ultrasound image to guide the HIFU ablation.

Patients with irregular vaginal bleeding need to undergo an endometrial biopsy to exclude endometrial lesions, and patients with severe anemia should be given an iron replacement or blood transfusion if the hemoglobin is less than 7 gm/dL. Even for those who have no contraindication for HIFU surgery, it is preferable to admit her to the hospital the day before the operation for preoperative preparation, signing consent, and communicating issues related to the HIFU surgery.

(b) Preoperative bowel preparation: Patients need strict preoperative diet preparation, usually 3 days before surgery; they should take a residue-free diet and easily digestible food, drink senna water to induce diarrhea 2 days before treatment, and full-liquid diet 1 day before treatment but no gas-producing foods, such as milk, soy milk, etc. Patients need to use compound polyethylene glycol electrolyte powder (or other cathartic drugs) to promote the elimination of intestinal contents in the afternoon on the day before treatment. The night before and the morning on the day of treatment, the enema exudates should be clear with no solid matters. During the bowel preparation, treatment, such as electrolyte supplementation and fluid replacement, can be given, particularly in older women or women with some medical illnesses.

(c) Skin preparation, degreasing, and degassing of the skin in the area within the acoustic pathway, including the skin below the navel, pubic symphysis, and perineal skin; no hair is left within the ultrasound energy pathway, and care should be taken not to create abrasions or wounds on the skin. Before treatment, further communication and psychological counseling with the patient will reduce their tension and anxiety.

14.1.2 Treatment

14.1.2.1   Administration of Sedation and Analgesia

The purpose of sedation and analgesia is to enable patients to tolerate any unpleasant surgical procedure, eliminate patients' anxiety and tension, and reduce the reaction to pain. It allows patients to maintain a certain level of consciousness to reflect the feelings correctly and respond to the doctor's and nurse's instructions during the surgery. During the operation, the patient's heart rate, blood pressure, respiratory rate, and blood oxygen saturation are monitored by an electrocardiogram monitor.

Many anesthetists have their protocols to provide sedation and analgesia according to their experience. They will use the same drugs according to their preference for sedation and analgesia. However, they usually tailor the drug according to the needs of patients and titrate the dosages based on her sedation level. In the absence of anesthetists, a similar program from different centers can be given to the patient as advised by their anesthesiology department. During the sedation and analgesia medication, closely observe the patient's heart rate, blood pressure, respiratory rate, and blood oxygen saturation.

14.2   Therapeutic Equipment

The USgHIFU treatment described in this book is based on a focused ultrasound tumor therapeutic system JC 200 model manufactured by Chongqing Haifu Medical Technology Co., Ltd. It operated with a treatment frequency of 0.94 MHz with a focal length of 138 mm. The HIFU tumor therapeutic system JC 200 is shown in Fig. 14.1. It has a transducer with a 20-cm diameter to produce ultrasound energy, with an ultrasound imaging probe (My-Lab70, Esaote, Italy) incorporated within the center of the transducer. The ultrasound probe enables real-time sonographic monitoring during HIFU ablation.

During the treatment process, the patient lies prone on the HIFU treatment bed, under conscious sedation (Fig. 14.2).

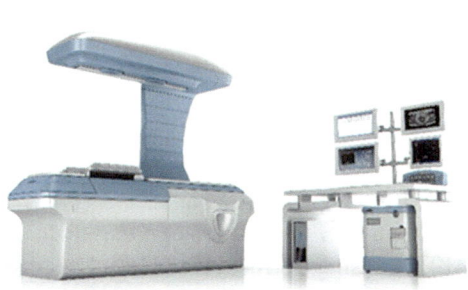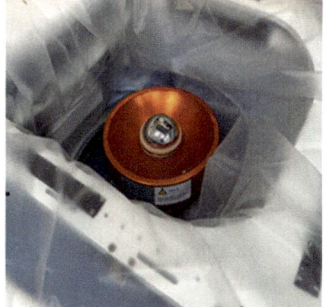

Fig. 14.1 The HIFU tumor therapeutic system JC 200. The ultrasound transducer and controller platform, with the ultrasound monitoring probe fixed at the center located under the treatment bed

Fig. 14.2 HIFU ablation of adenomyosis with a patient lying prone on the treatment bed. The HIFU transducer was mounted under the treatment bed, as shown

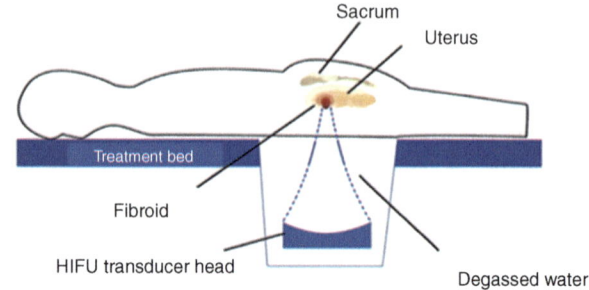

Fig. 14.3 JC 200 computer console to operate the USgHIFU ablation for adenomyosis

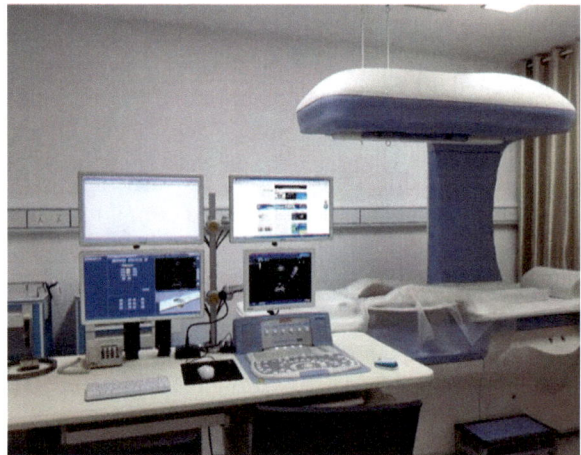

A urinary Foley catheter is required in the patient's bladder to control the bladder volume and to adjust the uterine position. The skin of the patient's abdomen is now placed in contact with cold (at 10 °C) degassed water. A computer console (Fig. 14.3) is to monitor the treatment by real-time ultrasound scan and to control the therapeutic ultrasound transducer platform for a six dimension movement.

With the six dimension movement of the transducer, together with the central ultrasound probe, the location, size, and shape of the uterus and the adenomyosis lesions are identified on the ultrasound image. A real-time ultrasound scan is to determine the location of the uterus in a sagittal view.

The following procedures will be performed for adenomyosis ablation.

1. Before the HIFU ablation, microbubble angiography with a microbubble contrast agent (SonoVue, Bracco, Italy) is performed before the start of treatment and at the end of treatment to assess the extent of the ablated area (Fig. 14.4). The ablation treatment can begin 10 min after the infusion of ultrasound microbubble contrast agent, to avoid HIFU causing microbubble-induced injury.
2. Before the start of the treatment, the sagittal plane of the uterus or adenomyoma is scanned; a treatment plan is made by dividing it into many slices with a thickness of 5 mm each from its left to the right ends.

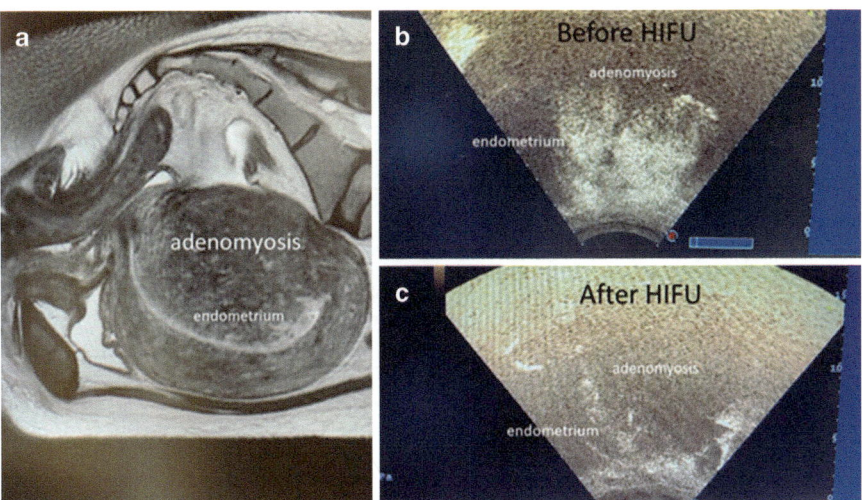

Fig. 14.4 (**a**) MRI image demonstrated posterior adenomyosis in the uterus; the endometrium was visible. (**b**) IV Infusion of microbubble before HIFU ablation, an ultrasound contrast agent, to visualize and estimate the sizes of the adenomyosis lesion. The endometrium was shown to be more intense perfused with microbubble (**c**) After HIFU ablation, non-perfusion areas of adenomyosis lesion can now be estimated, with the endometrium still intact, showing microbubble perfusion

3. Under the therapeutic parameters based on the locations, sizes, and vascularity of the adenomyosis lesions, the ultrasound energy emitted from the therapeutic ultrasound transducer passes through the skin into the body, focusing on the adenomyosis lesion through a pool of circulating cooled degassed water. The adenomyosis lesion on each slice should be ablated from the deep part before finally to the superficial part of the lesion, and this process is repeated slice by slice to achieve treatment of the entire adenomyosis lesion. The HIFU ablation can be guided by an MRI image incorporating into the real-time ultrasound image so that the target area can be easily visualized and provide more safety (Fig. 14.5).

4. Due to the fixed focal length and size of the focused ultrasound transducer, the HIFU ablation target may need to be adjusted by positioning a degassed water bag between the abdomen and the HIFU transducer. In this way, some superficial lesions can be reached.

5. During ablation, it is important is to establish a safe acoustic pathway without any gas bubble or small bowel within the pathway. By adjusting the size of the degassed water bag, increased filling of the bladder with normal saline or increased pressure on the abdomen by the ultrasound transducer or ultrasound probe; this can help to push the small bowel away from the front of the uterus, to establish a safe acoustic pathway, and to avoid bowel injury and damage to other non-target tissues.

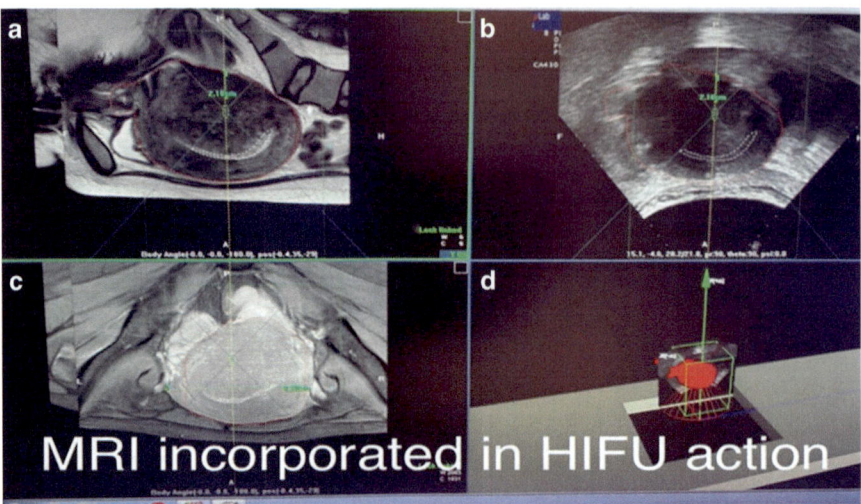

Fig. 14.5 The MRI image of the adenomyosis and its incorporation into the ultrasound image during HIFU ablation. (**a**) Sagittal MRI image with uterine and endometrial outlines marked out. (**b**) These MRI outlines were incorporated into the ultrasound image during HIFU ablation treatment. (**c**) Transverse MRI image in the pelvis (**d**) 3D positioning of the target lesion for easy location of the HIFU target

Fig. 14.6 Ultrasound monitoring of HIFU treatment with lesion showing gray-scale change during HIFU ablation

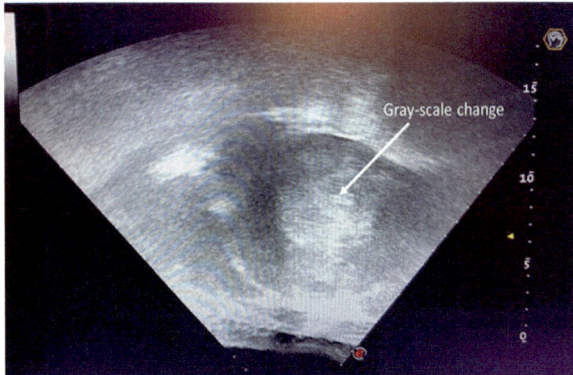

6. The ultrasound energy power used is adjusted to 300–400 W, with energy intermittently applied. Each energy exposure lasts for 1 second with a rest period of 3 seconds. HIFU sonication continues at a spot when a gray-scale change appears or up to a defined time of sonication (Fig. 14.6).

7. The target point of the focused ultrasound is to ablate the adenomyosis lesion slice by slice, and each time the focus is positioned with a safety margin of 1–1.5 cm from the uterine serosa and the endometrium. The ablation procedure starts at the central slice. When there is a significant increase in gray-scale change, the target focus will move to the next area, then the next layer for treatment, and the treatment is completed when the gray-scale change occurs in

each slice of the lesion to be ablated. The diagnostic ultrasound probe is used to monitor the gray-scale changes in the target lesion and the patient's movement, if any.

8. Cautions are taken to avoid sonication ablation close to the endometrium and serosa of the uterus. This protocol will help to minimize the thermal injury to the endometrium and surrounding tissues situated next to the uterus. During the HIFU procedure, the target location, energy power, sonication time, and treatment interval should be adjusted according to the patient's complaint or response. Any pain experienced by the patient at the time of treatment should alert the doctor of any potential risks of nerve or skin injury, with appropriate prompt management. Therefore it will reduce the risk of skin burns and nerve damage [2].

9. After the end of the HIFU procedure, the volume of the ablated lesion is roughly estimated by the non-perfusion volume during a repeat microbubble infusion, i.e., lesion areas not filled with contrast agents.

10. After the surgery, the patient should lie prone, and catheterization is maintained for another 1–2 h. The abdominal skin was given ice compress, if the patient is complaining of skin hotness. Other treatments, such as analgesic, antibiotics, and fluid replacement, if necessary, can be given. Keep observation of the patient's postoperative side effects closely for appropriate and timely treatment.

The patient can complete the treatment of HIFU in a relaxed and pleasant environment. The entire process does not create open wound or keyhole wounds, with no bleeding or general anesthesia, and the patient can mobilize immediately after HIFU treatment. After the patient finishes HIFU treatment, she is kept in the observation room for 1–2 h (non-inpatients) or stay in the hospital until the next day for observation. If the vital signs are stable and there is no obvious discomfort, they can be discharged home and leave the hospital.

References

1. Orsi F, et al. High-intensity focused ultrasound ablation: effective and safe therapy for solid tumors in difficult locations. Am J Roentgenol. 2010;195(3):W245–52.
2. Zhang L, et al. Ultrasound-guided high intensity focused ultrasound for the treatment of gynaecological diseases: a review of safety and efficacy. Int J Hyperth. 2015;31(3):280–4.

The Therapeutic Effect of HIFU on Adenomyosis

15

Mingzhu Ye

About 70% of patients with adenomyosis have clinical symptoms, including pain, such as dysmenorrhea, chronic pelvic pain, dyspareunia, and menstrual abnormalities as increased menstrual bleeding and prolonged menstrual period. It may also produce pressure symptoms due to the uterine enlargement caused by adenomyosis [1]. A large number of studies have also confirmed that adenomyosis can affect women's pregnancy and fertility, including subfertility and even infertility, as well as affect adverse obstetric outcomes, such as miscarriage, premature delivery, premature rupture of membranes, and also affect the treatment outcomes of in vitro fertilization [2–5]. These clinical symptoms are often the reasons for the patient's consultation visits. When evaluating the treatment effectiveness of adenomyosis, on the one hand, the safety of the method must be considered. On the other hand, the improvement of the above symptoms and obstetrics outcomes should also be evaluated. As a new treatment method for adenomyosis, we should consider HIFU, not only its non-invasive approach but also its safety and effectiveness. Here we summarize the efficacy of HIFU treatment for adenomyosis in this chapter.

15.1 Short-term Efficacy of HIFU in the Treatment of Adenomyosis

At present, the related researches on the efficacy of HIFU in the treatment of adenomyosis are mainly based on short-term efficacy. The relevant results suggest that HIFU treatment of adenomyosis can reduce the uterine volume and adenomyotic lesions in the short term and also effectively relieve the dysmenorrhea and heavy menstrual flow.

M. Ye (✉)
Department of Gynecology and Obstetrics, Third Xiangya Hospital of Central South University, Changsha, Hunan, China

Before HIFU is widely used in the treatment of adenomyosis, in order to study its safety, Yang et al. [6] performed HIFU ablation of diseased uteri in seven cases of adenomyoma at the time of open hysterectomy. They used a handheld HIFU transducer to ablate the uterus with focal adenomyosis. The histological examination of the ablated uterus showed coagulative necrosis at the ablated site of the adenomyoma. The boundary at the ablated area showed sharp demarcations between the damaged and the normal tissues, which proved that HIFU would be an effective method for the treatment of adenomyosis without damage to the surrounding normal tissue.

Since then, HIFU technology has begun to apply clinically for adenomyosis treatment. In 2008, Yoon et al. [7] reported a case of HIFU treatment for a 47-year-old patient with adenomyoma. During the 6–12 months follow-up, the patient had obvious improvement of her symptoms of dysmenorrhea and heavy menstrual flow, the quality-of-life (QOL) score after HIFU treatment improved significantly, and the size of the patient's uterus decreased by 35% 1 year after treatment.

With the increasing popularity of HIFU treatment to manage adenomyosis, many clinical studies had been published since then. Zhou et al. [8] reported on 78 cases of HIFU treatment in patients with adenomyosis, of which 69 patients were followed up for at least 18 months. Sixty-two patients were relieved of dysmenorrhea and menstrual disorders, but eight patients had relapsed symptoms. Lee et al. [9] reported the follow-up results of 346 patients with symptomatic adenomyosis who were treated with HIFU. They found that the proportions of uterine volume reduction at 3, 6, and 12 months after treatment were 43.99%, 47.01%, and 53.98%, respectively, and the severity of their symptoms reduced by 55.61%, 52.38%, and 57.98%, respectively. At the same time, the QOL score were 80.06%, 69.39%, and 85.07% at 3, 6, and 12 months during the follow-up. Also, Marques et al. [10] conducted a meta-analysis and systematic review of nine articles that reported clinical outcomes of HIFU treatment for adenomyosis. Of 729 patients, the great change in the uterine volume at 12 months was observed with a standard mean difference (SMD) = 0.85. It was also found that dysmenorrhea symptoms were significantly relieved at 3 months (SMD = 1.83) and 12 months (SMD = 2.37), and a significantly better QOL at 6 months (SMD = 3.0) and 12 months (SMD = 2.75) after treatment. These studies have confirmed that HIFU has a good short-term effect (tentatively about 1 year) on adenomyosis, especially for dysmenorrhea and abnormal menstruation.

15.2 Medium to Long-Term Efficacy of HIFU Treatment for Adenomyosis

Compared with the studies for the short-term efficacy of HIFU treatment for adenomyosis, studies for its long-term efficacy were few. In recent years, some studies have demonstrated not only the long-term efficacy of HIFU in treating dysmenorrhea and menstrual disorders of adenomyosis but also the effect of HIFU on pregnancy outcomes.

Shui et al. [11] reported 350 symptomatic adenomyosis patients treated with ultrasound-guided HIFU, of which 224 patients completed 2 years of follow-up. Among 203 patients with dysmenorrhea symptoms, after treatment, at 3 months, 1 year, and 2 years of follow-up, the remission rates of dysmenorrhea were 84.7%, 84.7%, and 82.3%, respectively, while in 109 patients with polymenorrhea at 3 months, 1 year, and 2 years of follow-up, their remission rates were 79.8%, 80.7%, and 78.9%, respectively, therefore indicating that HIFU treatment not only relieves the patients' dysmenorrhea and menstrual disorders in the short term after treatment but also have a long-term symptom relief effect. Liu et al. [12] reported the follow-up of 230 cases of symptomatic adenomyosis under HIFU treatment with ultrasound monitoring. A total of 208 out of the 230 patients had a median follow-up of 40 months (range 18–94 months). Of the 208 patients, 173 (83.2%) patients had a decrease in dysmenorrhea VAS scores, and 71% of whom had symptoms disappeared. The average dysmenorrhea score after treatment was significantly lower than before treatment. Thirty-seven patients had anemia due to increased menstrual flow before treatment, and their menstrual flow and hemoglobin returned to normal during the follow-up period. During the follow-up process, 45 (26%) of the 173 patients with dysmenorrhea symptoms improved after treatment was found to have relapsed. The median time to relapse was 12 months (range: 3–74 months).

In addition to the proven efficacy of HIFU treatment for adenomyosis, there were a few studies on the pregnancy status and outcome of patients after treatment. In theory, HIFU treatment should be the safest method for patients who wish to get pregnant. First, HIFU treatment is conducted under ultrasound or nuclear magnetic guidance, without radioactivity; secondly, HIFU treatment is precisely targeted to the lesion, without damaging the normal uterine tissue around the lesion, and can maximize the preservation of the integrity and function of the uterus. Unlike other interventional treatment, like uterine artery embolization (UAE), treatment does not affect the blood flow and function of the uterus and ovaries, so as to better protect the fertility of the patient.

Lee et al. [9] compared the anti-mullerian hormone (AMH) levels of 79 patients with symptomatic adenomyosis and uterine fibroids before HIFU treatment and 6 months after HIFU treatment. He found that there was no significant difference between the two, suggesting that HIFU treatment had no obvious impact on ovarian functions. Rabinovici et al. [13] reported a case of adenomyosis treated with MRgHIFU ablation. The patient had natural pregnancy 3 months after HIFU treatment. Ultrasound examination throughout the pregnancy period indicated normal fetal development and normal placental attachment. The patient had a vaginal delivery at full-term pregnancy, and yet the placenta was difficult to deliver after the birth of the baby. Manual removal of the placenta and exploration of the uterine cavity were performed. No serious complications occurred during and after delivery. Zhou [14] analyzed the pregnancy outcomes of 68 patients with adenomyosis who had fertility requirements after treatment with HIFU; 54 patients had a successful pregnancy with a median treatment to pregnancy time of 10 months. Among them, 20 patients had spontaneous abortions, 21 patients had delivered at full term with no uterine rupture, and all the newborns were normal. These preliminary results showed that HIFU treatment of adenomyosis improves patients' symptoms, without increasing complications of pregnancy and childbirth.

15.3   The Complications of HIFU Treatment

Despite the effectiveness and non-invasive nature of HIFU treatment for adenomyosis, it can have complications arising from its treatment. Therefore its operational safety is one of the main considerations when choosing this treatment method. Through much practice, it has been found that HIFU may have some adverse reactions during and after the treatment of adenomyosis. These include vaginal discharge, vaginal bleeding, and skin burn complications in the treatment area. Other adverse effects are abdominal pain; abnormal perineal, sacral, and lower limb pain or discomfort; urinary retention; hematuria; etc. Lastly, some rare complications also occur, such as abnormal kidney function, bowel injury, and even abdominal wall hernia [15, 16].

Feng et al. [16] conducted a retrospective study of 417 HIFU patients with adenomyosis and found that based on their results, ultrasound-guided HIFU is safe for the treatment of diffuse adenomyosis. Although the total pain complication rate during treatment was 92.3%, which is mainly related to pain experienced at the treatment area (80.1%) and sacral tail pain (55.6%) and skin burning pain (39.3%), etc. during the ablation treatment. According to the International Association of Interventional Radiology Severity Classification (SIR) standards [17], all were grade A or grade B, and no grade C or higher complications occurred. The safety analysis of 9988 cases of uterine fibroids and adenomyoma treated by Chen et al. [15] showed that in a total of 1062 patients, 1305 adverse reactions occur. Of the 1305 patients, 1228 were SIR class A and 45 cases SIR class B, 24 cases SIR class C, and the remaining 8 cases SIR class D. The more serious complications included three cases of acute renal insufficiency, two cases of bowel injury, and one case of long-term abdominal wall hernia. It can be seen that although HIFU treatment has more types of adenomyosis-related complications and a higher incidence, most of them are mild, and the incidence of serious complications is extremely low. Therefore, the HIFU treatment of adenomyosis still has high safety.

In summary, HIFU has good short-term and long-term effects on adenomyosis, with mild complications, and does not affect the fertility or pregnancy outcome after treatment. It is a safe and effective method to treat adenomyosis.

References

1. Gordts S, Grimbizis G, Campo R. Symptoms and classification of uterine adenomyosis, including the place of hysteroscopy in diagnosis. Fertil Steril. 2018;109(3):380–388. e1.
2. Matalliotakis IM, Katsikis IK, Panidis DK. Adenomyosis: what is the impact on fertility? Curr Opin Obstet Gynecol. 2005;17(3):261–4.
3. Maheshwari A, et al. Adenomyosis and subfertility: a systematic review of prevalence, diagnosis, treatment and fertility outcomes. Hum Reprod Update. 2012;18(4):374–92.

4. Juang CM, et al. Adenomyosis and risk of preterm delivery. BJOG Int J Obstet Gynaecol. 2007;114(2):165–9.
5. Younes G, Tulandi T. Effects of adenomyosis on in vitro fertilization treatment outcomes: a meta-analysis. Fertil Steril. 2017;108(3):483–490.e3.
6. Yang Z, et al. Feasibility of laparoscopic high-intensity focused ultrasound treatment for patients with uterine localized adenomyosis. Fertil Steril. 2009;91(6):2338–43.
7. Yoon S-W, et al. Successful use of magnetic resonance–guided focused ultrasound surgery to relieve symptoms in a patient with symptomatic focal adenomyosis. Fertil Steril. 2008;90(5):2018. e13–5.
8. Zhou M, et al. Ultrasound-guided high-intensity focused ultrasound ablation for adenomyosis: the clinical experience of a single center. Fertil Steril. 2011;95(3):900–5.
9. Lee J-S, et al. Ultrasound-guided high-intensity focused ultrasound treatment for uterine fibroid & adenomyosis: a single center experience from the Republic of Korea. Ultrason Sonochem. 2015;27:682–7.
10. Marques ALS, et al. Is high-intensity focused ultrasound effective for the treatment of adenomyosis? A systematic review and meta-analysis. J Minim Invasive Gynecol. 2020;27(2):332–43.
11. Shui L, et al. High-intensity focused ultrasound (HIFU) for adenomyosis: two-year follow-up results. Ultrason Sonochem. 2015;27:677–81.
12. Liu X, et al. Clinical predictors of long-term success in ultrasound-guided high-intensity focused ultrasound ablation treatment for adenomyosis: a retrospective study. Medicine. 2016;95(3):e2443.
13. Rabinovici J, et al. Pregnancy and live birth after focused ultrasound surgery for symptomatic focal adenomyosis: a case report. Hum Reprod. 2006;21(5):1255–9.
14. Zhou C. High-intensity focused ultrasound ablation technology to treat the efficacy of uterine adenomyosis and pregnancy outcome. Zunyi: Zunyi Medical College; 2017. p. 1-z.
15. Chen J, et al. Safety of ultrasound-guided ultrasound ablation for uterine fibroids and adenomyosis: a review of 9988 cases. Ultrason Sonochem. 2015;27:671–6.
16. Feng Y, et al. Safety of ultrasound-guided high-intensity focused ultrasound ablation for diffuse adenomyosis: a retrospective cohort study. Ultrason Sonochem. 2017;36:139–45.
17. Khalilzadeh O, et al. Proposal of a new adverse event classification by the society of interventional radiology standards of practice committee. J Vasc Interv Radiol. 2017;28(10):1432–1437. e3.

Adjuvant Therapy of HIFU Ablation for Adenomyosis

16

Mingzhu Ye

At present, many studies have confirmed that HIFU is a safe, effective, and non-invasive method for treating adenomyosis. Still, at the same time, we also realize that this HIFU treatment also has certain limitations. One of them is similar to all other uterine preservation treatment for adenomyosis; patients will face problems of poor results and recurrence. Clinical studies have confirmed that the effective rate of HIFU alone in treating adenomyosis is about 80%–90%, and there are still 10%–20% of patients whose symptoms do not improve significantly. Besides, there are still some patients with symptoms soon recur after treatment. Liu et al. [1] reported that 45 of the 173 patients with adenomyosis after HIFU treatment had symptoms recurred; the recurrence rate was about 26%, and the median time to relapse is 12 months.

In the same situation, when it faces the problems of poor treatment results and recurrence by conservative surgery for adenomyosis, some studies have demonstrated that adjuvant drug treatment can effectively reduce and delay the recurrence of symptoms of adenomyosis [2]. Also, some guidelines clearly state that in adenomyosis, long-term medical treatment is recommended to prevent the recurrence of symptoms after conservative treatment. Therefore, the need for long-term management of HIFU for adenomyosis has also been widely recognized in the treatment of adenomyosis.

At present, the long-term adjuvant treatment commonly used with HIFU to treat adenomyosis is mainly medical treatments, including mifepristone, gonadotropin-releasing hormone agonist (GnRH-a) and levonorgestrel-releasing intrauterine system (LNG-IUS), progesterone, etc. These medical treatments are described as follows:

M. Ye (✉)
Department of Gynecology and Obstetrics, Third Xiangya Hospital of Central South University, Changsha, Hunan, China

© The Author(s), under exclusive license to Springer Nature Singapore Pte Ltd. 2021
M. Xue et al. (eds.), *Adenomyosis*, https://doi.org/10.1007/978-981-33-4095-4_16

143

16.1 Mifepristone

Mifepristone is an estrogen and progesterone receptor antagonist that can inhibit follicular development and ovulation, inhibit the hypothalamic-pituitary-ovarian axis, and cause amenorrhea. At present, a few researchers have tried to combine mifepristone with HIFU to treat adenomyosis and achieved good results. Jiang et al. [3] compared the efficacy of HIFU alone and HIFU combined with mifepristone in the treatment of adenomyosis. Their results suggested that compared with before treatment, the degree of dysmenorrhea, menstrual flow, and the uterine volume were all decreased at 6 months after treatment. The total clinical effective rate of the combined treatment group was significantly higher than that of the HIFU alone group. Mao et al. [4] studied 100 patients with adenomyosis, who were randomly allocated into a HIFU-mifepristone study group and a HIFU control group and compared their clinical symptoms, uterine volume, and lesion size of the two groups before and after treatment. The results showed that the proportion of grade V to VI (severe) pain in all patients decreased from 22% before treatment to 7% at 12 months after treatment; the average uterine volume decreased by 18%, and the lesion volume decreased by 26%. Compared between the two groups, the dysmenorrhea remission rate of the study group after 6 months and 12 months of treatment was significantly higher than that of the control group, and the anemia remission rate of the study group was also significantly higher than the control group.

At present, the specific drug regimen of HIFU combined with mifepristone in the treatment of adenomyosis has different protocols reported in the literature. Many used mifepristone 12.5 mg taken daily from 1 to 2 months before HIFU treatment or starting from 1 to 5 days at the first menstrual period after HIFU treatment for 3 months.

16.2 Gonadotropin-releasing Hormone Agonist (GnRH-a)

GnRH-a is a synthetic hormone and endocrine drug, which can inhibit ovarian function but also bind to GnRH receptors in the pituitary, endometrium, myometrium, etc., and inhibit adenomyosis by exhausting its receptor. It can also reduce the blood supply to the uterus, reduce the volume of the uterus, improve the symptoms of dysmenorrhea and menorrhagia, etc. It is a commonly used conservative treatment for adenomyosis, and it is also used for long-term postoperative management.

In the treatment of adenomyosis, many studies have confirmed that HIFU combined with GnRH-a treatment can improve the therapeutic effect. Guo et al. [5] showed that HIFU treatment alone compared with HIFU combined with GnRH-a treatment; there is no significant difference in the efficacy at 1 month after treatment. Nevertheless, at 6 and 12 months after treatment, there was a significant improvement of dysmenorrhea, heavy menstrual flow, and lesion size reduction in the combined treatment group than the HIFU treatment alone.

Tan and Li [6] also compared the efficacy of HIFU alone and HIFU combined with GnRH-a in the treatment of adenomyosis. Eighty-four patients were randomized into two groups (42 patients each) and found that the total effective rate of the combined treatment group was 90.48% and the HIFU alone group 73.81%. The volume of the lesions in the two groups was significantly reduced at 1 month, 3 months, and 6 months after treatment, and the volume of the lesions in the combined treatment group at 3 months and 6 months was more obvious than that in the HIFU treatment group. All serum CA125, menstrual volume, and dysmenorrhea visual anolog scale (VAS) scores were significantly decreased after HIFU treatment. There was no statistically significant difference in adverse effects between the two groups during treatment.

At present, there is no standardization of GnRH-a usage for the treatment of adenomyosis after HIFU ablation. GnRH-a is generally given on the first day of the next menstrual period after HIFU treatment. Depending on the size of the uterus and the severity of symptoms, 4–6 courses of treatment are given. Besides, studies have confirmed that pre-treatment of adenomyosis with GnRH-a can improve the efficacy of HIFU treatment. Zhang et al. [7] confirmed that 1 to 3 courses of GnRH-a treatment before HIFU treatment of adenomyosis could obtain a larger ablation volume and effective ablation rate than the HIFU treatment group alone, and at 3 and 6 months follow-up, patients had a higher rate of symptom relief.

16.3 Levonorgestrel-Releasing Intrauterine System (LNG-IUS)

The LNG-IUS is also known as Mirena IUD, a new type of hormone-containing intrauterine birth control device, which can evenly release the high-efficiency progesterone, levonorgestrel (LNG), which can provide a long-term conservative medical treatment for adenomyosis. It is also one of the commonly used adjuvant treatments after HIFU ablation for adenomyosis.

Huang et al. [8] studied 42 cases of HIFU treatment, 44 cases of LNG-IUS intrauterine placement, and 43 cases of adenomyosis treated with HIFU combined with LNG-IUS. They found that the uterine volume, dysmenorrhea score, menstrual volume, and endometrial thickness were significantly reduced in the HIFU with LNG-IUS group at 3 months and 6 months after treatment than the other two groups. Wu et al. [9] studied 15 cases of adenomyosis patients treated with HIFU combined with LNG-IUS and 15 cases of HIFU alone and found that compared with the same group before treatment, the dysmenorrhea score and the uterine fibroid symptom-quality of life (UFS-QOL) score were significantly reduced; when compared with the HIFU alone group, the dysmenorrhea score was significantly decreased at 3, 6, and 12 months, the UFS-QOL score and serum CA125 level also significantly decreased at 6 and 12 months after HIFU combined with LNG-IUS treatment. Therefore, compared with HIFU alone, HIFU combined with LNG-IUS is more effective in improving patients' dysmenorrhea and improving quality of life. At present, the specific protocol of HIFU combined with Mirena for the treatment of adenomyosis has not standardized. Most of the Mirena IUD placement is at 2–5 days after the first or third menstrual period after HIFU treatment.

16.4   Other Single Adjuvant Therapy with HIFU

There are a few papers that reported other adjuvant treatments associated with HIFU ablation. Luo et al. [10] studied the efficacy of HIFU combined with gestrinone in the treatment of adenomyosis. In their study, the efficacy of HIFU alone and HIFU combined with gestrinone in 30 patients with adenomyosis was analyzed. Among them, patients in the combined treatment group started taking gestrinone 2.5 mg, two times weekly after HIFU ablation. After taking it for 3 months, the follow-up results showed that the improvement in menstrual flow and dysmenorrhea scores at the 6 and 12 months after treatment was statistically significant. Compared with the HIFU control group, the raised hemoglobin level of the combined treatment group was statistically significant 6 months after treatment. There are also studies suggesting that HIFU combined with absolute alcohol injection [11]; Chinese herbal medicine [12] can also improve the efficacy of HIFU in its treatment of adenomyosis. Even more, Hou et al. [13] had studied HIFU combined with metformin in the treatment of adenomyosis. The improvement of the menstrual flow and pain, as well as the reduction of serum inflammatory factors, was significantly better than the HIFU treatment group alone.

16.5   Combined Adjuvant Therapies with HIFU

In addition to the single adjuvant treatment approach in the above studies, some studies reported the use of combined adjuvant treatment together with HIFU for treating adenomyosis, and its effect is obvious. Sun et al. [14] reported the result of 142 patients with adenomyosis treated with HIFU combined with GnRH-a and LNG-IUS. They were followed up for 5 years. At 12 months after treatment, the size of the uterus shrinks obviously with an average reduction of about 45% and then slightly increases and stabilizes at a reduction rate of about 35%. The volume of uterine adenomyosis, dysmenorrhea scores, and menstrual volume also had similar declines. During this long-term 5 years follow-up, the recurrence rate of dysmenorrhea and menorrhagia are also low, approximately 5.68% and 7.91%, respectively. It is suggested that HIFU combined with GnRH-a and LNG-IUS is a safe and effective method for the treatment of adenomyosis. Yang et al. [15] also treated 466 patients with HIFU combined with GnRH-a and LNG-IUS. After treatment, both the dysmenorrhea and menstrual symptoms were significantly relieved, the uterine volume basically returned to normal, and the serum CA125 level also dropped to normal. Ye et al. [16] retrospectively analyzed the efficacy of HIFU ablation, HIFU combined with GnRH-a, HIFU combined with LNG-IUS, and HIFU combined with GnRH-a + LNG-IUS in treating dysmenorrhea of adenomyosis and found that long-term efficacy of HIFU combined with LNG-IUS + GnRH-a in the treatment of dysmenorrhea of adenomyosis is significantly better than that of HIFU alone and HIFU combined with GnRH-a. The difference is statistically significant.

Regarding HIFU and its combination therapy, there is currently no unanimous opinion. The present experience showed that (1) if the patient's symptoms are mainly dysmenorrhea, and the uterus enlargement is less than 2 months of pregnancy, and there is no fertility requirement in a short period, LNG-IUS can be placed after the menstruation 3 months after HIFU treatment; (2) if the uterus is more than 2 months of pregnancy, with heavy menstrual flow, but without fertility requirements within a short period, it is recommended to give GnRH-a treatment for 4–6 months after HIFU treatment. LNG-IUS can be placed 1–2 months before GnRH-a is stopped; (3) for patients with obvious uterine enlargement and fertility requirements, 4–6 courses of GnRH-a treatment is given further to reduce the size of the uterus after HIFU treatment, and patients should be encouraged to get pregnant soon a few months after HIFU and GnRH-a treatment.

In summary, after HIFU treatment of adenomyosis, long-term management should be maintained for symptomatic relief. Various methods and drugs have been used as adjuvant treatments for adenomyosis treated with HIFU, and studies have shown that combined treatment methods often have better efficacy in both short and long term than HIFU treatment alone. However, at present, there is still a lack of agreed standards and specific treatment plans for adjuvant treatments, because patients have a different extent of diseases, associated conditions, and variations of symptoms. When selecting appropriate adjuvant treatment, it is necessary to follow the individualized principle according to the specific situation of the patient. Hopefully, in the future, large-scale multicenter prospective studies can be conducted to confirm the efficacy of HIFU in the treatment of adenomyosis, to clarify the indications of various adjuvant treatments, and guide a better clinical practice.

References

1. Liu X, et al. Clinical predictors of long-term success in ultrasound-guided high-intensity focused ultrasound ablation treatment for adenomyosis: a retrospective study. Medicine. 2016;95(3):e2443.
2. Wang P-H, et al. Comparison of surgery alone and combined surgical-medical treatment in the management of symptomatic uterine adenomyoma. Fertil Steril. 2009;92(3):876–85.
3. Jiang D, Liu X. High-intensity focused ultrasound combined with mifepristone to treat uterine adenomyosis and the effects on pain. Chin Commun Phys. 2019;30:23.
4. Mao Shihua TX, Ling F, Zongguo T, Tao Z, Lian Z. High-intensity focused ultrasound combined with mifesterone to treat uterine adenomyosis. Chin Family Planning Obstet Gynecol. 2014;6(5):29–31.
5. Guo Q, et al. High intensity focused ultrasound treatment of adenomyosis: a comparative study. Int J Hyperth. 2018;35(1):505–9.
6. Tan Yutao LZ. High-intensity focused ultrasound noninvasive therapy combined with gonadotropin release hormone agonists to treat uterine adenomyosis – an observation. Chin Mater Child Health. 2019;34(20):4811–5.
7. Xiao-Ying Z, et al. Effect of pre-treatment with gonadotropin-releasing hormone analogue GnRH-α on high-intensity focussed ultrasound ablation for diffuse adenomyosis: a preliminary study. Int J Hyperth. 2018;34(8):1289–97.
8. Huang Xia YB, Hong Z, Denghua J. The clinical efficacy analysis of high-intensity focused ultrasound in combination with Mirena IUD in the treatment of uterine adenomyosis. Pract Gynaecol Endocrinol Elect J. 2018;15:33–5.

9. Wu Ziyu PZ, Xiuping L, Yueyue D, Mingjie J. Clinical observation of high-intensity focused ultrasound in combination with LNG-IUS treatment of uterine adenomyosis. Shandong Med. 2018;58(3):65–7.
10. Luo Shuang WY, Jia H. Evaluation of the efficacy of high-intensity focused ultrasound ablation combined Gestrinone to treat uterine adenomyosis. Chongqing Med. 2018;47(2):170–2.
11. Ding G. Clinical study of high-intensity focused ultrasound combined with aqueous ethanol to treat uterine adenomyosis. Zhonghua Fu Chan Ke Za Zhi. 2017;51(9):643–9.
12. Xiangjie L Clinical study of ultrasound ablation combined herbal analgesic capsules for the treatment of uterine adenomyosis. New Town Medical College; 2015.
13. Hou Y, et al. Combination therapeutic effects of high intensity focused ultrasound and metformin for the treatment of adenomyosis. Exp Ther Med. 2018;15(2):2104–8.
14. Haiyan S, et al. High-intensity focused ultrasound (HIFU) combined with gonadotropin-releasing hormone analogs (GnRHa) and levonorgestrel-releasing intrauterine system (LNG-IUS) for adenomyosis: a case series with long-term follow up. Int J Hyperth. 2019;36(1):1179–85.
15. Yang X, et al. Combined therapeutic effects of HIFU, GnRH-a and LNG-IUS for the treatment of severe adenomyosis. Int J Hyperth. 2019;36(1):485–91.
16. Ye Mingzhu DX, Xiaogang Z, Min X. High-intensity focused ultrasound ablation combined GnRH-a and LNG-IUS in the treatment of uterine adenomyosis. Chin J Obstet Gynecol. 2016;5:1–9.

The Pregnancy Outcomes After Uterine Preservation Surgery and HIFU Treatment for Adenomyosis

17

Can Xie

The clinical manifestations of adenomyosis are complicated, and there are many clinical treatments, but there is no single method that can resolve all the problems of adenomyosis. It is especially so for the treatment of patients with adenomyosis with infertility. Chen [1] emphasized that the treatment of adenomyosis should pay attention to the surgical techniques and the combined application of other treatment methods. Therefore, it is believed that the same principle should be applied for patients with adenomyosis and infertility, focusing on combined therapy.

At present, there is no consensus on the treatment of adenomyosis that will improve and preserve the patient's fertility. Gonadotropin-releasing hormone agonist (GnRH-a) long-term therapy combined with assisted reproduction has become the most commonly used method in clinical practice. Due to the complex etiology of adenomyosis, there are no recommendations to the surgical indication for patients with adenomyosis and infertility. Lang [2] proposed that in selected patients, surgical treatment can improve fertility outcomes. Patients with uterine adenomyosis can be selected for surgery if they meet the following criteria: (1) Ineffective medical treatment or other medical conditions that patients are not suitable for medical treatment. (2) Before assisted reproductive technology (ART) treatment, the uterus is large with focal lesions (adenomyoma). (3) No significant decrease in uterine or adenomyosis volume after GnRH-a pretreatment before ART or repeated embryo implantation failure.

C. Xie (✉)
Department of Gynecology and Obstetrics, Third Xiangya Hospital of Central South University, Changsha, Hunan, China

17.1   Uterine Preservation Surgery

Uterine preservation surgeries are divided into adenomyosis resection (adenomyo-mectomy) for localized adenomyosis and volume reduction surgery for diffuse adenomyosis. Resection of adenomyoma can remove the localized diseased tissue from the normal myometrium, which causes less damage to the surrounding normal myometrium. However, for diffuse adenomyosis, the volume reduction surgery requires the removal of a large piece of adenomyosis tissue, including intertwined healthy myometrial tissue. Thus the damage to the myometrium would be great. Whether conservative uterine preservation surgery should be performed on patients with adenomyosis is still controversial. The adenomyosis lesion is characterized by the aggressive growth of the adenomyosis involving the inner myometrial layer. While the surgeon attempts to remove the lesion completely, it may also cause the removal of a whole myometrial layer and damage the underlying endometrium, resulting in a large defect of the uterine myometrium and a uterus with weakened uterine wall, thereby increasing the risks of uterine rupture during pregnancy and labor. A serious complication, such as placental implantation, may also occur. When the adenomyoma is relatively focal, the pregnancy rate and live birth rate of patients after adenomyoma resection are higher. When the lesion is diffuse, it is necessary to analyze the situation and carefully evaluate the possible advantages and disadvantages of the surgery. Also, surgery should not only deal with the adenomyosis itself but the associated pelvic endometriosis, deep infiltrating endometriosis (DIE), uterine fibroids, etc. The extent and type of surgery may affect the outcomes of fertility and pregnancy.

17.2   Pregnancy Outcomes After Surgical Treatment of Adenomyosis

In 2018, "Endometriosis Management Guidelines" from the French Association of Obstetricians and Gynecologists and the French National Health Administration pointed out that the operation of uterine adenomyoma with a diameter of less than 6 cm did not improve the outcomes of fertilization, pregnancy, and birth rate. However, there is no related report of operations for adenomyosis with a diameter of more than 6 cm [3]. Therefore, this guideline did not recommend surgical intervention for patients with larger adenomyoma. However, there are also different opinions. Some small clinical studies had shown that patients with pre-operative infertility could have natural pregnancies after surgery, indicating that excision of uterine adenomyosis can play a role in promoting pregnancy. Since the first report of adenomyosis resection in 1990, more than 2000 cases of such patients have been reported worldwide in 2018, of which 89.8% were reported by the Japanese [4]. The emphases of the surgical methods were on the techniques of resection and suture. They are focal lesion resection, wedge resection, H-type resection, three-lobe suture, U-shaped suture, etc. Osada et al. [5] reported that 26 patients with fertility requirements had 16 successful pregnancies after resection of adenomyosis lesions,

14 full-term deliveries, and no uterine rupture. Saremi et al. [6] performed wedge-shaped resection of 103 cases of adenomyosis with severe symptoms (46 of which were infertile); 21 cases tried natural pregnancy after surgery, and 7 of them were successful. However, the number of these reported cases is limited, and the selection criteria are different. Clinically, there is a huge difference in the severity of adenomyosis combined with infertility, then who can benefit from the surgery remain controversial? Therefore surgery needs to be assessed carefully. Kishi et al. [7] analyzed multiple factors relating to the outcomes after conservative surgery. They found that the pregnancy rate of patients aged ≥40 years was significantly lower than that of patients under 39 years old (3.7% vs. 41.3%). For young patients, surgery may bring benefits. When the patient complains of severe pain symptoms, ineffective or failed medical treatment, complicated endometriosis, DIE in the pelvis, subfertility or repeated pregnancy failure, etc., if surgical treatment is to be performed, the patient should be carefully assessed and counseled for appropriate fertility surgery, emphasizing the implementation of individualized treatment.

The postoperative use of ART may increase the pregnancy rate. Still, age is an important factor affecting the pregnancy rate in patients with adenomyosis, especially those over 40 years old. The clinical value of conservative surgery is limited.

17.3 Pregnancy Outcome After Surgery for Focal Adenomyoma Is Superior to Diffuse Adenomyosis

Research data from Tsui et al. [8] showed that the pregnancy rate after resection of focal adenomyoma was 48.2% to 77.5%, the successful delivery rate was 26.8% to 69.0%; but, the pregnancy rate after diffuse adenomyosis is about 30% to 40%; nearly 1/3 to 1/4 of patients had a successful delivery. In the study of Grimbizis et al. [9], the pregnancy rate after complete resection of adenomyosis was 60.5%; the pregnancy rate after partial resection of the lesion was about 46.9%. Tan et al. [10] conducted a systematic review of 1396 cases of infertile women with focal and diffuse adenomyosis in 18 studies. The results showed that after focal adenomyoma resection, the average pregnancy rate, live birth rate, and miscarriage rate were 49.1%, 38.6%, and 27.6%; after surgical resection for diffuse adenomyosis, the above rate was 38.5%, 31.3%, and 16.2%. Therefore, for suitable cases, fertility-sparing surgery is effective in increasing the pregnancy rate, and the benefit after surgery for focal adenomyoma is superior to that of diffuse adenomyosis.

17.4 Surgery or Combined Drug Treatment Can Improve the Pregnancy Rate of Patients

Wang et al. [11] reported that resection of adenomyosis combined with GnRH-a in patients with adenomyosis and infertility could significantly prolong the period of symptom remission compared with GnRH-a alone. The 3-year cumulative pregnancy rate was high [46.4% (13/28) vs. 10.8% (4/37), P = 0.002], and the 3-year cumulative successful delivery rate is high [32.1% (9/28) vs. 8.1% (3/37), P = 0.022].

17.5 Limitations of Conservative Surgery to Preserve Fertility

Surgical treatment of adenomyosis can improve fertility in some patients, but it also has limitations. Some normal myometrial tissues are missing after part of the adenomyosis is removed, and the normal myometrial tissue of the uterus is reduced during pregnancy, which can easily lead to miscarriage and premature delivery. Moreover, it is difficult to grasp the balance between removing the lesions as much as possible and maintaining the morphological integrity of the uterus. Conservative uterine surgery may lead to the damage of the uterine structure and the reduction of the uterine volume after the operation. A long period of contraception after surgery may further delay the timing of pregnancy. Besides, the probability of pregnancy complications during pregnancy increases, affecting live births. Uterine rupture is a complication of pregnancy and delivery after uterine surgery. In recent years, there were reports of uterine rupture during pregnancy after surgical excision of adenomyosis. Liu et al. [12] reported 114 cases of adenomyosis excision, of which 68 cases had pregnancies after the surgery, and 3 cases (4.4%) of them had ruptured uterus in pregnancy. Uncertainty in the extent of resection for diffuse adenomyosis may result in excessive resection of adenomyosis and the normal myometrium, resulting in a weak muscle layer, which becomes a high-risk factor for uterine rupture during pregnancy.

17.6 HIFU Treatment of Adenomyosis

HIFU is an emerging local non-invasive treatment method developed by combining the use of ultrasound in medicine with modern engineering technology. Ultrasound has characteristics, such as directivity, penetrability, and tissue sound absorption. HIFU uses these ultrasound characteristics and the biological effects of HIFU on ablating lesions. It accurately focuses the ultrasound energy emitted by the ultrasound transmitter onto the lesion in the body to destroy the lesion without damaging the surrounding normal tissues. The principle of HIFU's destruction of the lesion tissue is related to a series of biological effects of ultrasound. The most important of these is the thermal effect. HIFU can instantaneously raise the temperature of the lesion tissue at the focused site to above 60 ° C, thereby causing irreversible coagulative necrosis of the tissue. In addition, when the ultrasonic energy concentrates on the microbubbles developed from the heated up tissue, the microbubbles can be disintegrated, thereby instantaneously generating biological effects, such as cavitation effects resulting in high temperature and high pressure, which also play an important role in HIFU treatment. Also, the mechanical effect and dispersion effect of ultrasound certainly play an important role, and Yang et al. [13] had confirmed that HIFU could also improve and raise the specific and non-specific immunity of the treated areas, thereby killing the diseased cells through the immune response.

17.7 The Impact of HIFU on the Reproductive Functions

In an early study, Yang et al. [14] performed HIFU ablation to the uterus of seven patients at open hysterectomy for adenomyosis. After removing the uterus, specimens were taken for pathological examination. Coagulative necrosis was found in smooth muscle cells, glandular cells, and interstitial cells of the adenomyoma. It provided a theoretical basis for the clinical application of HIFU in the treatment of adenomyosis. In 2006, Rabinovici et al. [15] reported a case of successful treatment of adenomyosis with MRI-guided HIFU. However, there has been a concern that because of the lack of a lesion boundary in adenomyosis, then the heat conduction can be relatively diffused and easy to cause the damage to the uterine myometrium and endometrium adjacent to the lesion, thereby affecting the patient's fertility. Therefore, for women with fertility requirements, HIFU was once contraindicated for the treatment of adenomyosis. However, more and more studies suggested that women who had HIFU ablation could also conceive naturally [15, 16]. Therefore, in 2009, the Food and Drug Administration (FDA) changed the absolute contraindication to the relative contraindication for patients with fertility demand to receive HIFU treatment.

Furthermore, some studies also showed that HIFU treatment has no adverse effects on pregnancy and newborns [15, 16]. At present, the safety of HIFU in the treatment of adenomyosis has been recognized. HIFU treatment under real-time ultrasound monitoring can accurately ablate adenomyosis lesions, minimize damage to normal uterine tissues, and create conditions for a successful pregnancy after treatment.

17.8 Pregnancy Outcomes After HIFU Treatment in Patients with Adenomyosis

To some patients with adenomyosis who have fertility requirements, HIFU, as an emerging treatment method, has a strong advantage in maintaining the integrity of the uterus. Using ultrasound focusing on ablating adenomyosis lesions, it can restore the anatomy of the uterus and improve the immune microenvironment, and the pregnancy rate has increased after HIFU treatment. Zhou [17] reported 68 cases of adenomyosis treated with HIFU. Among them, 62 were diffuse, and 6 were focal adenomyosis. There were 59 pregnancies in 52 patients after HIFU ablation treatment for adenomyosis, and the median pregnancy time after treatment was 10 months (range: 1-31 months). Among them, 21 had delivered at full term, including 17 cesarean sections and 4 vaginal deliveries. Two pregnancies were ongoing at the time of reporting; there were 31 abortions, including 20 spontaneous abortions and 11 induced abortions. Wang et al. [18] 2017 analyzed the pregnancy outcomes of 20 patients with adenomyosis who were successfully conceived after receiving HIFU ablation. The pregnancy to treatment time was from 1 to 23 months, with an average of 8.75 (± 6.23) months. Of the 20 patients, 18 were naturally conceived and 2 through ART. All patients had no serious complications during pregnancy. Eleven patients had cesarean sections, including one case of premature delivery, one case placenta previa, and nine cases selected cesarean section. All patients who had delivered had no complications, such as threatened uterine rupture or uterine rupture during delivery. Among the 20 patients, 3 were patients with primary infertility, and they had delivered at full term successfully. Luo et al. [16] studied 38 cases of adenomyoma patients who had fertility requirements and treated with HIFU ablation. A total of 15 patients out of the 38 patients were successfully conceived naturally after treatment. The average conception rate was 39.5%, and the conception time was 6 to 24 months. Among them, seven patients had delivered with three cesarean sections and four vaginal deliveries. Despite previous HIFU ablation, no obvious uterine abnormality was found during the cesarean sections. There were no uterine ruptures during pregnancy and childbirth. For the seven deliveries, the placenta detached spontaneously, and the uterus was well-contracted. The color Doppler ultrasound examination of the uterus also showed well involution with no abnormalities after 42 days of delivery. Tang et al. [19] analyzed the pregnancy outcomes of 30 patients with adenomyosis treated with HIFU and found that within 1 year after treatment, 24 of these 30 patients had a successful pregnancy and the pregnancy success rate was 80% (24/30). Among the 24 patients with a successful pregnancy, 18 cases (75%) and 6 cases (25%) underwent normal vaginal delivery and cesarean section, respectively.

From the above studies, we conclude that HIFU treatment is a safe and effective treatment for patients with adenomyosis and fertility requirements. HIFU treatment can improve their pregnancy rate, pregnancy outcome, and the pregnancy of patients with previous adverse obstetrical history. HIFU treatment of adenomyosis does not affect the patient's mode of delivery; thus patients with HIFU treatment can choose vaginal delivery without increasing the risks of complications during delivery. From the various reports in the literature, the best treatment to pregnancy interval can be shortened to 6-12 months after HIFU treatment.

17.9 Comparison of Pregnancy Outcomes of HIFU and the Conservative Surgery for Adenomyosis

It is still controversial whether the conservative surgical treatment of adenomyosis with uterine preservation can benefit patients who have fertility requirements. For some suitable patients, surgery can increase pregnancy rates and improve pregnancy outcomes. However, it must be targeted at patients with individualized analysis of their situation, e.g., a focal lesion, failed medical drug treatment, failed IVF-ET, and young patients with associated pelvic endometriosis or disorders; surgical treatment may then be beneficial. The time of contraception after surgery is much longer, because it needs time to allow the uterine wound to heal. Nevertheless, there is still a risk of recurrence of the adenomyosis during contraception. Even after successfully pregnant, patients still have the risks of premature delivery, miscarriage, and uterine rupture during pregnancy and childbirth. Therefore, the indications for surgery have to be well-balanced of the pros and cons. As a new treatment for adenomyosis, HIFU treatment has only a limited number of studies. However, from the analysis of clinical data currently available, HIFU treatment can significantly improve the fertility and pregnancy outcomes. The increase in pregnancy and childbirth rate is no less than that of surgical treatment. Because HIFU treatment is a non-invasive treatment without any wounds, it therefore would not damage the integrity of the uterus and possibly not associate with postoperative pelvic and abdominal adhesions. HIFU treatment guarantees an intact structure of the uterus, thus it allows a shorter treatment to pregnancy interval time after HIFU treatment. It is another advantage that makes HIFU a preferred option for patients who have fertility requirements.

References

1. Chen C. Several problems that should be paid attention to in the course of uterine adenomyosis diagnosis and treatment. Chin J Pract Gynaecol Obstet. 2017;33(2):134–6.
2. Lang J. Several problems with uterine adenomyosis. Chin J Pract Gynaecol Obstet. 2017;33(2):129–33.
3. Li Xia YH, Wenxuan H, Wei C, Yumin Z, 2018 French Association of Obstetricians and Gynaecologists/French National Health Service. Endometriosis management guide. Chin Pract Gynecol Obstet. 2018;34(11):1243–6.
4. Xu B. The management status and prospect of uterine adenoid disease combined infertility. China Family Planning Obstet Gynecol. 2019;4:3.
5. Osada H. Uterine adenomyosis and adenomyoma: the surgical approach. Fertil Steril. 2018;109(3):406–17.
6. Saremi A, et al. Treatment of adenomyomectomy in women with severe uterine adenomyosis using a novel technique. Reprod BioMed Online. 2014;28(6):753–60.
7. Kishi Y, Yabuta M, Taniguchi F. Who will benefit from uterus-sparing surgery in adenomyosis-associated subfertility? Fertil Steril. 2014;102(3):802–807. e1.
8. Tsui K-H, et al. Conservative surgical treatment of adenomyosis to improve fertility: controversial values, indications, complications, and pregnancy outcomes. Taiwanese J Obstet Gynecol. 2015;54(6):635–40.
9. Grimbizis GF, Mikos T, Tarlatzis B. Uterus-sparing operative treatment for adenomyosis. Fertil Steril. 2014;101(2):472–487. e8.
10. Tan J, et al. Reproductive outcomes after fertility-sparing surgery for focal and diffuse adenomyosis: a systematic review. J Minim Invasive Gynecol. 2018;25(4):608–21.
11. Wang PH, et al. Is the surgical approach beneficial to subfertile women with symptomatic extensive adenomyosis? J Obstet Gynaecol Res. 2009;35(3):495–502.
12. Liu Wei ZM, Yanyan Y. Study on pregnancy after uterine adenoidectomy in infertility patients. China Medical Guide. 2017;14(8):92–5.
13. Yang R, et al. Effects of high-intensity focused ultrasound in the treatment of experimental neuroblastoma. J Pediatr Surg. 1992;27(2):246–51.
14. Yang Zhu CY, Lina H, Zhixuan W. High intensity focused ultrasound first study of pathological changes in adenomyosis in human body. J Clin Ultrasound Med. 2003;5(2):65–7.
15. Rabinovici J, et al. Pregnancy and live birth after focused ultrasound surgery for symptomatic focal adenomyosis: a case report. Hum Reprod. 2006;21(5):1255–9.

16. Luo S, et al. Pregnancy outcome after high intensity focused ultrasound (HIFU) treatment for patients with adenomyosis. Chongqing Med. 2014;4:454–455, 458.
17. Chunyan Z High-intensity focused ultrasound ablation to treat uterine adenomyosis - its effects and pregnancy outcome. Zunyi Medical College; 2017. p. 1-z.
18. Wang Zhi ZM, Li C, Yongbin D, Yu X. Observation of pregnancy outcome after high intensity focused ultrasound treatment in patients with adenomyosis. Chongqing Med. 2017;46(18):2506–8.
19. Tang B. Evaluation of the effect of high-intensity focused ultrasound ablation on adenomyosis patients with fertility requirements. J Contemp Med. 2019;17(19):76–7.

Conclusion

18

Felix Wong

Adenomyosis is due to the invasion or presence of endometrial glands in the uterine myometrium accompanied by hyperplasia and hypertrophy of the surrounding muscle cells, forming either a diffuse or localized lesion. The pathogenesis was discussed in detail in the previous chapters. While the incidence of adenomyosis varies according to the diagnostic criteria and population, it is about 20% to 30% of women.

The clinical symptoms of adenomyosis are dysmenorrhea, heavy menstrual bleeding, infertility, and other diseases related-symptoms. These symptoms are presented in detail in Chaps. 5, 6, and 7. Today, the diagnosis of adenomyosis is confirmed by ultrasound or/and magnetic resonance imaging (MRI). Computerized tomography (CT) is insensitive compared with MRI scan. Besides, CT scan has undesirable radiation effects. MRI gives a very good resolution of various tissue layers, besides its advantages of being non-technical dependence, unaffected by bowels, bladder sizes, and surrounding tissues. Its disadvantage is the high cost that not all patients can afford for a routine examination. The ultrasound scan is still commonly used for the diagnosis of adenomyosis. It can provide a cost-effective approach to diagnose adenomyosis. However, ultrasound diagnosis depends on the skill and technique of ultrasound scanning by the operators, not to say the quality of the machine. The criteria to diagnose adenomyosis by ultrasound imaging and MRI had been elaborated in the related Chaps. 8 and 9.

Medical or surgical treatments for adenomyosis are to relieve the pelvic pain and dysmenorrhea, to reduce the heavy menstrual bleeding and anemia, and to improve fertility. Sometimes a combination of pain killers, hormones, and surgery is necessary to improve the treatment result. Pretreatment diagnosis is necessary to allow starting treatment early and using the appropriate treatment. Symptomatic treatment

F. Wong (✉)
School of Women's and Children's Health, The University of New South Wales, Sydney, NSW, Australia
e-mail: fwong3@hotmail.com.hk

based on clinical awareness or infertility is often practiced, because firstly, adenomyosis involves younger reproductive-aged women. However, the result of medical or surgical treatment is not effective up to patients' satisfaction. Both surgical complications and side effects of the long-term medications are often not welcomed by patients or even doctors. There are currently no international guidelines to follow for surgical or medical treatment of adenomyosis. As many patients in the reproductive age group may suffer from adenomyosis, there is a growing consensus that they need long-term management plans, including pain and bleeding control, fertility preservation, and pregnancy assistance.

As the first-line treatment, patients with adenomyosis can benefit from medical treatment with progestin, gonadotropin-releasing hormone agonists (GnRHa), nonsteroidal anti-inflammatory drugs (NSAIDs), levonorgestrel intrauterine system (LNG-IUS), and combined oral contraceptives, but only for a short period till they wish to get pregnant. The medications and usage of drug treatment are similar to those for endometriosis, with a slightly different focus on various medications as listed in the relevant Chap. 10. Nevertheless, medical treatment is not without side effects, and they all have adverse impacts on fertility. Sometimes they may not be able to control the symptoms, which may get severe as the adenomyosis progress. Also, for patients starting drug treatment, they should be followed for at least 1–3 months to monitor the occurrence of adverse reactions and deal with them accordingly. For older women, many only benefit from a hysterectomy, yet not all wish to accept this surgical treatment. Conservative surgery is then used to manage patients with adenomyosis. The surgical treatment will hopefully relieve symptoms and severity and preserve fertility desire. The indications of conservative surgery should include (1) dysmenorrhea and hypermenorrhea that failed to control with medication and (2) intolerability or contraindications to long-term medication. For older patients who do not have fertility requirements, they can choose a total hysterectomy; for younger patients who desire to preserve fertility or the uterus, they can select conservative surgery, that is, fertility-sparing operations.

The purpose of the conservative surgery is to remove the lesion, preserve the uterus, and even preserve fertility. Conservative surgery for adenomyosis is divided into (a) adenomyomectomy for focal adenomyosis, (b) cytoreductive surgery for diffuse adenomyosis, and (c) endometrial ablation or resection. However, conservative surgery for adenomyosis is difficult to perform and may not achieve a good result. Although conservative surgery is effective in relieving symptoms, the recurrence of symptoms after surgery is high, mainly due to the presence of residual adenomyosis tissue, which is difficult to remove completely. The wound healing is also poor compared with myomectomy. Therefore the risk of uterine rupture (6.8%) after conservative surgery is much higher than that for uterine fibroid removal (about 0.26%). Although hysterectomy is still the ultimate treatment for women with severe symptoms, conservative surgical options should be offered for women who wish to maintain fertility. The limitation of conservative surgery and its approach is discussed in Chap. 11.

Nowadays, we have benefited the shifting from minimally invasive surgery to non-invasive focused ultrasound surgery. However, conservative fertility-sparing surgery for adenomyosis is more effective by open surgery because of the technical difficulty of surgery. This book has elaborated on a new non-invasive treatment approach for adenomyosis. It is the high intensity focused ultrasound surgery (HIFU) ablation surgery for adenomyosis.

The "high intensity focused ultrasound surgery (HIFU)" is the application of an ultrasound-guided HIFU (USgHIFU) or MRI-guided HIFU (MRgHIFU) ablation to solid tumors, e.g., liver cancer, pancreatic cancer, bone tumors, soft tissue tumors, and benign uterine diseases. The principle of HIFU treatment is to focus the ultrasound energy within the body after safely penetrating the body tissue. The main therapeutic mechanisms include thermal, cavitational, and mechanical effects. The principles and therapeutic protocols of HIFU ablation treatment for adenomyosis are discussed in Chap. 13.

HIFU ablation has lately been used to treat focal adenomyoma or diffuse adenomyosis. The use of the two HIFU treatment systems, MRgHIFU and USgHIFU, as well as the HIFU treatment result are elaborated in Chaps. 14 and 15 in the book. The purpose of HIFU ablation treatment is to ablate and reduce the sizes of lesions, control the growth, relieve dysmenorrhea, and improve clinical symptoms. However, many kinds of research on the efficacy of HIFU treatment for adenomyosis are mainly based on short-term efficacy, and new data regarding adjuvant therapy to HIFU ablation is elaborated in Chap. 16. The long-term management after HIFU treatment for adenomyosis is mainly drug therapy, and related studies have confirmed that HIFU combined with GnRHa, with LNG-IUS, and HIFU or GnRHa + LNG-IUS in the treatment of dysmenorrhea had long-term efficacy and were significantly better than HIFU alone. Also, the recurrence rate was significantly reduced.

Finally, the comparative result of pregnancy outcome after myomectomy and HIFU ablation for adenomyosis is discussed in Chap. 17.

To summarize this new treatment approach, we know that HIFU is not perfect in the treatment of adenomyosis. Because HIFU is a non-invasive treatment, patients accept it more readily than conventional medical and surgical treatments, which have undesirable side effects and complications. Despite early favorable treatment results, the recurrence rate is worth closely examined. A combination with drug treatment to control the symptoms appears to be preferable. However, this will continue to impact on the fertility in this group of reproductive-aged women, especially those with fertility demand. Based on the pathogenesis of adenomyosis, the preservation of the endometrium by HIFU ablation will certainly end with some degrees of recurrence. Therefore for the treatment of adenomyosis, the key issues are (1) early diagnosis of adenomyosis by imaging technology to offer prompt surgical treatment, such as HIFU ablation, to reduce the extent and symptoms of adenomyosis; (2) early pregnancy, if applicable, might help to reduce the adverse impact of the later development of adenomyosis; (3) more research in the etiology, development, and treatment of adenomyosis may shed more light on the future management of adenomyosis.

GPSR Compliance

The European Union's (EU) General Product Safety Regulation (GPSR) is a set of rules that requires consumer products to be safe and our obligations to ensure this.

If you have any concerns about our products, you can contact us on ProductSafety@springernature.com

In case Publisher is established outside the EU, the EU authorized representative is:

Springer Nature Customer Service Center GmbH
Europaplatz 3
69115 Heidelberg, Germany

Batch number: 10091879

Printed by Printforce, the Netherlands